Resistance Band Workout

Resistance Band Exercises for Strength Training

(Quick and Easy Resistance Band Exercises for Regain Muscle Safety)

Danny Schreier

Published By **Jessy Lindsay**

Danny Schreier

Resistance Band Workout: Resistance Band Exercises for Strength Training (Quick and Easy Resistance Band Exercises for Regain Muscle Safety)

ISBN 978-1-9990334-2-2

No part of this guidebook shall be reproduced in any form without permission in writing from the publisher except in the case of brief quotations embodied in critical articles or reviews.

Legal & Disclaimer

The information contained in this book is not designed to replace or take the place of any form of medicine or professional medical advice. The information in this book has been provided for educational & entertainment purposes only.

The information contained in this book has been compiled from sources deemed reliable, and it is accurate to the best of the Author's knowledge; however, the Author cannot guarantee its accuracy and validity and cannot be held liable for any errors or omissions. Changes are periodically made to this book. You must consult your doctor or get professional medical advice before using any of the suggested remedies, techniques, or information in this book.

Upon using the information contained in this book, you agree to hold harmless the Author from and against any damages, costs, and expenses, including any legal fees potentially resulting from the application of any of the information provided by this guide. This disclaimer applies to any damages or injury caused by the use and application, whether directly or indirectly, of any advice or information presented, whether for breach of contract, tort, negligence, personal injury, criminal intent, or under any other cause of action.

You agree to accept all risks of using the information presented inside this book. You need to consult a professional medical practitioner in order to ensure you are both able and healthy enough to participate in this program.

Table Of Contents

Chapter 1: Warm-Up and Stretching

Before beginning resistance band carrying sports activities, properly warming up your muscle mass and joints to keep away from harm is important In this financial disaster, you'll examine greater about smooth heat-up moves and stretching sports to prepare your frame.

First, the economic wreck explains why warming up and stretching will become more vital as you age. Your muscle tissues get tighter, and joints get stiffer with age, so that you want to counteract this. Then, the bankruptcy explores unique warmness-up wearing sports to increase your heart charge, enhance blood go along with the waft on your muscles, and put together your frame for movement.

Lastly, the financial catastrophe takes you via head-to-toe stretching exercises to decorate flexibility on your palms, legs, lower again, and center. Following the step-with the useful resource of-step commands and images, you'll lightly stretch all of the foremost muscle groups in band training.

With right warmness-up and stretching, your body can be prepared to take at the resistance band bodily sports correctly.

Importance of Warm-Up and Stretching

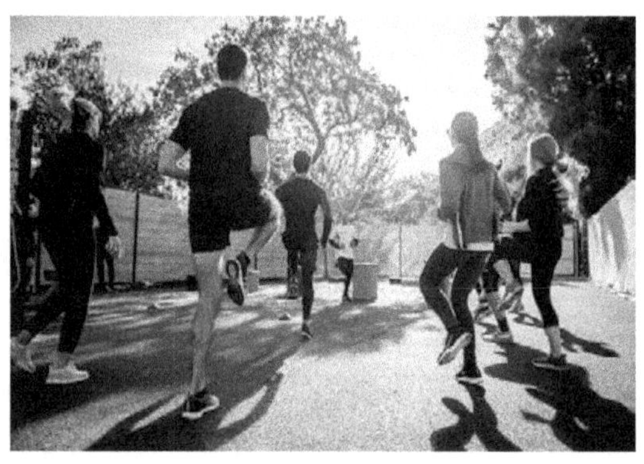

Warming up earlier than resistance band workout is critical for seniors to boom blood float and put together the body for education. Light aerobic hobby, like walking, gently increases core frame temperature, developing flow and providing extra oxygen and nutrients to muscle groups for power production. It heats muscles and joints, making tissues greater pliable and conscious of resistance bands, and joint lubrication is advanced, permitting smoother movement. Warming up primes the cardiovascular tool and reduces the possible chance of damage.

Dynamic Warm-Ups Enhance Mobility

Performing dynamic heat-up bodily video games incorporating frame weight movements is notable for seniors to prepare for resistance band sporting activities. Dynamic heat-u.S.A.Involve squats, lunges, presses, and extraordinary beneficial sporting sports without out of doors resistance. Moving the frame through these motions enables activate and heat up the unique muscle groups targeted throughout band schooling commands.

Going via the gathering of each exercising rehearses proper strategies, appealing the only of a type motor patterns. It specializes in coordination and neural activation, priming the nervous tool and muscle groups to carry out the moves as quickly as you have delivered resistance from the bands. The dynamic drills take the body through a comfortable variety of motion, lubricating joints and improving mobility earlier than training.

Dynamic heat-u.S.A.Gently enhance coronary coronary heart price and middle body temperature due to the fact the maximum essential muscle groups are placed via their paces. It circulates blood waft to working regions, developing oxygenation and vitamins to muscle groups. The raised temperature makes muscle mass more pliable and aware about resistance. Joints additionally advantage from mild mobilization.

The key's performing managed multi-joint movements at an clean tempo. Eventually, greater repetitions can be completed to build up amount and growth center temperature. Movement need to be ache-loose through the entire sort of movement. The essential effect is rehearsing the exercise movements, activating muscular tissues, elevating coronary heart price, and enhancing mobility in training for real resistance schooling. Dynamic drills set the frame up for achievement.

Stretching for Flexibility and Recovery

Dedicated stretching after warming up is also alternatively useful for seniors using resistance bands. Stretching muscle tissues even as warmth makes tissues extra elastic and pliable, lowering natural muscle stiffness that could in any other case limit mobility. Warm muscle tissues can be lengthened in addition with out pressure or micro-tearing.

Taking joints via a comfortable entire variety of motion for the duration of stretching improves flexibility. Seniors can characteristic and pass through wider levels pain-unfastened. Enhanced flexibility permits you to move approximately each day sports extra without problems, and the joints advantage from being mobilized thru lengthened positions.

Stretching after sports lets in flush out metabolic waste like lactic acid that builds up in muscle tissues in some unspecified time in the destiny of exertion. Flushing waste merchandise enables exercise restoration with the aid of reducing pain and fatigue. Stretching even as warmness additionally will increase blood flow, delivering clean oxygen and vitamins to rush up muscle restore.

Maintaining flexibility and joint variety of movement thru everyday stretching makes schooling safer and permits save you harm, particularly for seniors. Age-related stiffness can be mitigated to maintain mobility. Keeping tissues limber reduces the opportunity of pulls, strains, or tears in the route of exercising routines. Stretching moreover protects the joints.

The secret is preserving relaxed stretches for extended times while breathing deeply, allowing muscle tissue to release constructed-up anxiety and re-set up most useful resting length. A appropriate rule of thumb is 30 seconds in line with stretch, that specialize in vital muscle corporations. Stretches must no longer purpose ache. Light tension that dissipates is proper.

Stretching Lowers Heart Rate and Tension

In addition to the bodily benefits, stretching after resistance wearing events additionally has intellectual and emotional advantages for seniors. Slow static stretches paired with deep diaphragmatic breathing assist lower coronary coronary heart charge after exertion. This returns the cardiovascular tool to a snug u . S . After being active subsequently of the workout.

Deep respiration at the equal time as retaining stretches additionally lowers blood stress as oxygen saturation stabilizes. Breathing techniques promote reduced arousal, lowering pressure hormones like adrenaline that building up during exercise and facilitating everyday calmness.

The mixture of static stretching and respiration stimulates the parasympathetic anxious machine, which controls the frame's rest and recuperation. Activating the parasympathetic response initiates muscular relaxation and quietens the mind. Stretching is a valuable cool-down signal to the body that the exertion is over and it's time to recover.

Holding stretches calls for inner cognizance on body alignment and proper form, growing more thoughts-frame recognition, which you carry over into every day existence. Releasing regions of amassed tension via targeted stretching creates right away release. This body popularity helps manipulate strain.

Seniors would possibly possibly discover innovative relaxation and centered respiratory at some point of stretching after resistance schooling nearly meditative. Moving through clean stretches with cause at the equal time as controlling breath price and depth has a centering effect. The stretches can be savored and feature a re-centering ritual post-exercising.

Tailoring the Warm-Up for Seniors

When planning a warm-up normal for seniors using resistance bands, tailoring the sports activities to because it must be prepare their our our our bodies for exercising with out overdoing it's far crucial. The warm-up must bear in mind the bodily boundaries that frequently consist of age to get the blood flowing and muscular tissues heated earlier than schooling efficiently.

Low-intensity aerobic movements like walking mixed with gentle stretching art work properly for older adults. For human beings with mobility troubles, the exceptional and snug-up moves can be completed seated to prompt the muscle groups with out bearing weight. Seniors new to training will gain from an prolonged warmness-up section with extra sets of motion drills for the principle muscle companies.

This heat-up affords more time to regularly growth the frame temperature earlier than jumping into the exercising. Specific stretches based on preferred age-associated postural styles and which purpose areas wherein seniors often have tightness may be blanketed. The secret is customizing the fine and comfortable-as a lot as address person skills and needs. You can heat up nicely for workout and reduce damage risks with the proper coaching.

Warm-Up Exercises

When making plans your warm temperature-ups, the bodily sports need to set off muscle organizations, mobilize joints, increase coronary coronary heart rate, beautify balance, and top the mind-body connection. Certain warmth-up sports activities are specifically well-suitable for seniors that optimize exercising average overall performance and safety. Warm-up wearing occasions for seniors encompass:

1.   Walking

Walking is one of the best and first-rate warm-up carrying events for seniors. Light cardiovascular sports activities like strolling lightly improve body temperature and get blood circulating to the running muscle mass. The progressed blood flow sends extra oxygen and vitamins to the muscle corporations that need it for strength manufacturing. Walking is low impact and adjustable in depth. Seniors can display their tempo and exertion diploma to live in a solid location. Those with boundaries can select out seated table sure cycling as an alternative.

2.   Dynamic Stretching

Dynamic stretching is likewise an terrific choice for senior warm temperature-ups. Dynamic stretches comprise taking joints via managed tiers of movement the use of most effective body weight resistance. Examples like leg swings, knee will boom, torso twists, and arm circles actively stretch most important muscle agencies. The movements are multi-planar, improving mobility on all planes. Dynamic stretches lightly start the notable and comfortable-up way before consisting of resistance bands. A controlled shape prevents overstretching.

three. Low-Intensity Squats and Lunges

Squats, lunges, presses, and different not unusual resistance band sporting activities can be included at lower intensities into the great and relaxed-up recurring. Using lighter bands or frame weight for 10-15 repetitions of essential physical video games executed with the proper approach, attractive high movers mimic the exercising. The awareness is on quality repetitions and mind-muscle connection, top notch-tuning the neuromuscular device.

4.   Balance Exercises

Challenging balance is every special super warm-up addition for seniors. Exercises like heel-toe stand, ahead/backward weight shifts, lateral side steps, and unmarried-leg balances lightly track proprioceptive structures. This light stability paintings engages stabilizers at the identical time as warming up the center and ankles. Movements can be finished with hand useful resource if desired. Balance improves posture and coordination.

five.   Breathing Exercises

Breathing bodily games are frequently not noted but offer intellectual warmth-usafor seniors. Taking 2-3 mins for deep, managed diaphragmatic respiratory turns on the parasympathetic anxious machine, reducing strain hormones and clearing the thoughts in coaching for schooling. Long, normal exhales reason rest in advance than exertion. This breathwork additionally can be performed seated.

Light Static Stretching

Light static stretching can be included on the end of the high-quality and comfy-as a great deal as deal with notoriously tight areas earlier than along with resistance.

Hamstrings, chest, hip flexors, and shoulders often benefit from short static holds of 15-30 seconds. This stretching expands the kind of motion and forestalls overstretching on the same time as using bands. Stretches have to not reason ache.

How Long Should Seniors Do Warm-Up Exercises?

The heat-up duration want to be prolonged for seniors who want extra time elevating center body temperature and lubricating joints in advance than progressing to schooling. The tempo also may be slowed with extra cardio sets if important. Adjustments ensure seniors are bodily and mentally organized.

Proper sequencing of these warmth-up wearing activities optimizes outcomes. Light cardio and mobility art work need to be carried out earlier than muscle activations for pliable tissues. The intensity builds up step by step by using manner of the usage of layering in dynamic and static drills earlier than shifting to resistance. Breathwork closes the recurring. This go with the flow makes the maximum of the overall ordinary performance.

Stretching Routines

Proper stretching after resistance schooling is critical for seniors to maintain joint health and versatility. Dedicated stretching exercises that take muscle groups via a whole form of motion provide complete-body benefits. Here are 12 powerful stretches that may be delivered to relax-downs:

Head Tilt

This stretch goals anxiety in the neck muscle mass. Here's the manner to do it:

1.   Start with the useful resource of fame tall with a right upright posture.

2.   Gently tilt your head inside the direction of one shoulder until you experience a moderate stretch up the aspect of the neck.

3.   Don't overdo the tilt - a moderate stretch sensation is proper.

four.   Hold this position for at least 30 seconds, respiratory deeply.

five.   Repeat on the other facet.

6.   Repeat as typically as you may.

Shoulder Box

This stretch mobilizes the shoulders and opens the chest. You can do it as follows:

1.   Start with the useful resource of extending your palms right now out to the edges at shoulder pinnacle, palms going thru down, developing a discipline shape with the hands.

2.   Draw massive backward circles with both arms concurrently.

3.   Circle for as a minimum 20 seconds.

4.   Reverse the path.

five.   Repeat as frequently as possible.

Moving the shoulders thru the ones big rotational levels of movement lubricates the shoulder joints.

Gas Pedal

The fuel pedal stretch dreams tightness in the front of the hip and thigh. You can without trouble do the fuel pedal stretch as follows:

1.   Sit tall in a chair.

2.   Extend one leg right away out in the front of you.

3.   Bend the other knee and region the foot throughout the thigh of your directly leg.

four. Reach in advance and clasp the bent leg close to the shin.

five.   Gently press the bent leg down within the course of the floor until you revel in a slight stretch inside the hip flexor of your right now leg.

6.   Hold for a couple of minutes, then transfer legs.

7.	Do it as commonly as feasible.

Side Bend

This stretch lengthens the obliques alongside the factor ribs. Here are the stairs to comply with while doing side bends as a senior:

1.	Stand with toes hip-width aside.

2.	Interlace your palms above your head, absolutely extending your arms.

3.	Lean your torso to 1 issue, reaching your hands over in the path of your toes, preserving your fingers prolonged overhead.

4.	A mild stretch want to be felt along the aspect frame.

5.	Hold for a few moments, then repeat on the alternative element.

6.	Repeat a few times.

Tennis Watcher

The tennis watcher stretch opens the chest and the front shoulders. Follow these steps to do the tennis watcher for seniors:

1.   Stand straight away with particular posture.

2.   Inhale slowly thru your nose as you switch your head as a ways left as snug without stress.

3.   Exhale through your mouth and preserve this function in brief, feeling the stretch for your neck muscles.

4.   Inhale lightly thru your mouth as you slowly turn your head to the proper.

5.   Exhale thru your mouth and keep this function.

6.   Repeat turning your head element to element as favored.

Lying Knee to Chest

This stretch goals the hip flexors and gives decrease lower back consolation. It additionally decompresses the spine.

1.   Lie to your lower back and hug one knee into your chest until you revel in a moderate stretch within the the front of your hip and thigh.

2.   Keep the alternative leg prolonged at the ground.

3.   Repeat collectively with your other leg.

4.   Repeat as desired.

Chapter 2: Upper Body Workouts

By now, you've stretched your muscle tissues and gotten your blood pumping. Now, you ought to positioned your better frame muscle organizations to artwork. This bankruptcy teaches you the manner to get toned and bolstered from your neck on your torso.

The financial disaster starts offevolved offevolved with key arm-strengthening wearing occasions the use of resistance bands. You'll be amazed how running your biceps and triceps improves each day responsibilities like carrying groceries or yard art work. This financial disaster walks you through every step.

You may discover the manner to artwork to your shoulders and pinnacle returned, that is for wonderful posture and to avoid hunching.

Furthermore, this economic catastrophe specializes in exercising the chest and middle muscle groups. A sturdy middle builds stability to hold you regular in your ft. You'll experience proud seeing the definition to your chest all over again.

By the surrender of the economic catastrophe, your top body will experience greater toned and capable after the workout. Read on to start sculpting your hands, shoulders, chest, and another time. Upper body electricity makes the whole lot from circle of relatives chores to gambling together collectively along with your grandchildren less difficult.

Arm Strengthening Exercises

Great arm-strengthening sports to add to a senior resistance band recurring encompass:

Bicep Curls

Bicep curls are an effective resistance band exercising for strengthening the the the front of the better palms. Here is a way to do them:

1.   Start with the aid of repute on the middle of the band with feet hip-width apart and take one result in every hand.

2.   Have your hands saved by way of way of the usage of your facet with the arms beforehand-coping with.

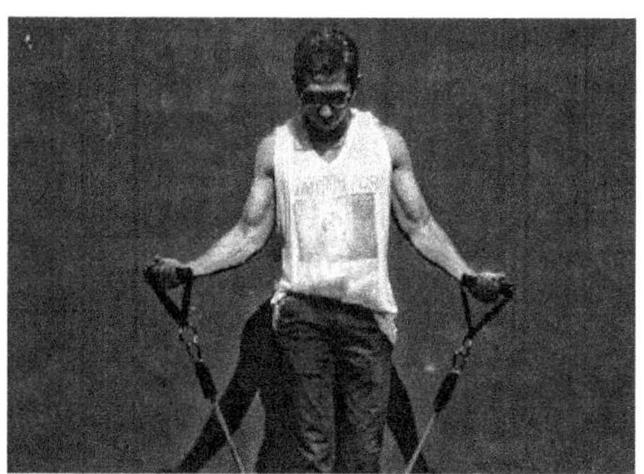

three. Take a deep breath at the identical time as preserving your lower lower back immediately. Squeeze your biceps as you bend your elbow inside the direction of you.

4.   Focus on keeping your elbows near the frame at a few level inside the movement to isolate the biceps nicely.

5.   Continue curling up until your fingers almost obtain your shoulders if cushty, squeezing the biceps at the top.

6.   Exhale and lower your fingers slowly and controlled.

7.   Repeat for 10-15 controlled repetitions, the usage of excellent shape to keep normal anxiety at the biceps.

8.   Do 2-three sets resting among.

Tricep Extensions

Stand in the middle of your resistance band with ft hip-width apart, and place one foot inside the middle of the band.

1.   Bring your palms inside the returned of your head, collectively with your elbows pointed within the course of the ceiling.

2.   Keep your pinnacle fingers though and stuck in place next on your head.

3.   Slowly straighten one arm once more and down in an arc shape.

four.   Only move the forearm, retaining the upper arm desk sure.

5.   Straighten the arm absolutely, pause, and move back to the start characteristic.

6.   Repeat this arc movement 10-12 instances.

7.   Switch and carry out 10-12 repetitions on the opportunity arm.

eight. Keep your elbows pointed up and glued subsequent for your head.

nine.   Use managed movement focusing on the triceps.

10.   Avoid swinging or the use of momentum.

eleven.   Exhale as you straighten your arm again, inhale as you come.

12.   Complete 2-3 sets with 30-60 seconds rest among.

Upright Rows

1.   Stand inside the middle of the band, toes hip-width apart.

2.   Grip the band with an overhand grip, and your hands some inches apart.

3.   Let your fingers increase down in the the front of your thighs.

four. Engage the pinnacle decrease again muscle groups.

five.   Exhale and pull your arms immediately up in the course of your chin.

6.   Keep your palms extended sooner or later of the movement.

7.   Bring your shoulder up.

eight. Inhale and slowly lower the band.

9.   Control the movement up and down.

10.   Repeat 12-15 instances with well form.

11.   Keep your better body though, and avoid swinging.

12.   Use the returned muscles to boost the band.

Front Raises

1.   Stand in the center of the band, feet hip-width apart.

2.   Arms are down with the aid of way of facets, palms going through once more.

3.   Slightly bend your elbows.

four.   Engage the center muscle mass.

five.   Raise each hands in the front to shoulder height.

6.   Raise palms in a managed motion.

7.   Keep a slight elbow bend at some point of.

8.   Raise fingers to eye stage if snug.

nine.   Pause in quick on the top.

10.   Slowly lower your arms decrease once more to the begin function.

eleven.   Repeat a managed beautify and lower at least 10 instances.

12.   Maintain suitable posture throughout.

Bent Over Rows

1.	Stand at the center of the band, ft hip-width apart.

2.	Bend beforehand at the hips to a 45-diploma bend.

3.	Keep your again immediately, now not round.

4.	Engage the center muscle companies.

5.	Extend your palms down closer to the floor.

6.	Initiate the row by way of the usage of squeezing the shoulder blades together.

7.	Pull your elbows up and reduce again, bringing the bands in your chest.

eight.	Keep your elbows tucked close to the edges.

9.	Bring your shoulder up.

10.	Stop for a second and convey the bands for your beginning function slowly.

11.   Control the movement up and down.

12.   Repeat severa times.

13.   Complete 2 units with a rest in amongst.

Overhead Presses

1.   Sit or stand maintaining the band at shoulder pinnacle.

2.   Keep your elbows bent at 90-diploma angles.

3.   Palms face ahead, with the band near your ears.

4.   Engage your middle muscle groups.

five.   Exhale and press your palms upward, straightening your elbows.

6.   Fully increase your fingers overhead with arms ahead.

7.   Pause in short at the top position.

8.   Inhale and slowly decrease your fingers once more to shoulder top.

nine.   Keep a mild bend in the elbows at the bottom.

10.   Repeat the clicking and decrease it for 10-12 managed times.

Reverse Flies

1.   Stand at the band center along with your fingers extended in front.

2.   Palms face every one-of-a-type, and your knees are smooth.

three. Maintain a slight bend within the elbows.

four. Initiate via squeezing the shoulder blades collectively.

5.   Pull the bands up and out to the edges in an arc motion.

6.   Lead along with your elbows, preserving them bent.

7.   Bring your shoulder up.

8.   Pause, then go back to the start feature.

nine.   Control the motion up and down.

10.   Repeat for 10 controlled instances.

11.   Focus on the use of your yet again muscle tissue.

12.   Start mild, then growth band resistance through the years.

thirteen.   Targets better all over again and shoulders.

It's vital to provide your muscle companies a rest day among resistance band arm workout sports to allow for healing and restore. Seniors want initially 1-2 devices of 10-15 repetitions for every exercising, 2-three instances per week. Increase the intensity step by step over numerous weeks using heavier resistance bands, together with a 2d set, and doing more repetitions constant with set. Proper vitamins with adequate protein consumption additionally permits seniors gain muscle.

Shoulder and Back Workouts

Front increases, lateral increases and upright rows referred to above also can exercising your shoulder and decrease again. You can improve your shoulder and lower again with those greater resistance band workout routines for seniors:

Shoulder Presses

1.   Stand with ft hip-width apart on the middle of the band.

2.   Raise every arms to shoulder peak at ninety-degree angles.

Chapter 3: Lower Body Workouts

This chapter specializes in your legs, glutes, and hips, the muscle mass that keep you upright and transferring. You'll begin with leg strengthening sporting sports to sculpt your quads, hamstrings, and calves. With those bodily games, you regain the strength for sports activities like mountain climbing stairs without difficulty or on foot simply. Resistance bands upload the right task for wonderful outcomes.

Balance is important as you age, so that you will observe unique exercises to beautify balance. Using the band, you'll development from standing on one foot to dynamic stances. Before you recognize it, you'll revel in regular and assured for your toes yet again.

Also, this financial disaster focuses on the glutes and hips. Weak hips and glutes can throw off your whole lower body alignment, major to pain. You will discover the manner to prompt these muscle tissues with bridging carrying sports, clamshells, and different key movements.

By the end of the chapter, your entire lower body will experience more resilient, out of your hips for your ankles. Read on and sculpt your leg, glute, and hip muscle groups. Strong lower frame muscles make ordinary sports a breeze.

Leg Strengthening Exercises

Maintaining sturdy, useful legs is significantly crucial to maintain mobility and independence as you age. Your legs let you perform endless each day sports activities, from taking walks the canine to mountaineering stairs to standing up from a chair. However, muscle businesses and strength decline through the years if not properly exercised. Hence, resistance bands are very beneficial for seniors seeking out an powerful manner to decorate their legs without heavy weights or machines.

Bands will permit you to load and pork up leg muscle mass in a controlled manner with out placing immoderate-impact forces on developing older joints. When blanketed successfully right into a senior fitness regular, resistance band leg sporting activities can beautify strength to maintain an lively manner of life.

Before leaping into leg sporting sports activities, continuously warm up first via taking walks or marching in region for as a minimum five-10 mins to increase blood go together with the go with the flow to the decrease frame. When performing the physical video games, waft slowly through a whole, pain-unfastened variety of motion for every rep, retaining off compromised shape. Focus on proper technique, posture, and respiratory. Allow a rest day amongst band leg physical games to provide the muscle organizations adequate restoration time. Gradually building up resistance with the useful resource of the usage of thicker bands over the years.

Banded Squats

They beautify the glutes, quads, and hamstrings. You can do them thru following the steps underneath:

1.   Stand along with your toes hip-width aside at the middle of the resistance band.

2.   Engage your center muscle businesses and keep your chest lifted.

3.   Initiate movement thru manner of sending the hips lower lower returned as although sitting in a chair.

four. Bend your knees and slowly move down until your thighs are parallel to the ground; if in a position.

five.   Make tremendous your knees stay in line over your feet all through the movement. Do no longer allow the knees cave inward.

6.   Keep your weight allocated gently among every feet.

7.	Reach your glutes yet again as you squat down.

8.	Keep your heels planted.

9.	Press lightly through your heels and midfoot to stand and move returned to the beginning function.

10.	Repeat controlled squat down and arise for 10-15 repetitions.

11.	Use lighter resistance to recognition on form earlier than growing band anxiety.

Side Leg Raises

Targets outer thighs and gluteus medius. Here are the stairs to conform with:

1.	Secure your resistance band to a robust object at the hip to ankle stage.

2.	Stand sideways with the band below the internal foot and hold onto a guide, like a chair, if desired.

3.	Maintain an upright posture with engaged center muscle companies.

4. Keeping the status leg barely bent, slowly improve the alternative leg right now out to the component.

5. Raise the lifted leg best approximately 2-three feet a long way from the standing leg.

6. Do now not lean your torso or pelvis sideways, and maintain your hips degree.

7. Hold in quick at the pinnacle, then slowly lower your leg. Return on your beginning function regularly with manipulate.

8. Complete 10 managed repetitions, then switch sides and carry out on the opposite leg.

Standing Leg Curls

Works hamstrings and glutes of the returned leg. Here's the way to do fame leg curls:

1. Stand upright, shielding a resistance band securely in each fingers.

2.   Step one foot onto the center of the band together together with your hands prolonged down thru your hips.

three. Shift your weight barely onto the the front bending leg.

four. Keep the decrease lower back leg extended proper now within the lower back of the frame with the knee absolutely prolonged - this is the going for walks leg.

5.   Start the motion thru slowly bending the the front knee at the identical time as simultaneously curling the again leg up through manner of using flexing the knee.

6.   Squeeze your glutes and hamstrings as you pull your heel towards your hips.

7.   Slowly lower over again to the beginning role with manipulate.

eight. Complete 10-12 repetitions, then switch legs and repeat at the alternative leg.

nine. Maintain an upright posture; do not lean in advance.

Seated Leg Extensions

This exercising objectives the quadriceps. Here are the steps to comply with:

1.   Sit tall close to the give up of a resistance band together along side your legs prolonged and one foot placed thru a loop inside the band.

2.   Keep your decrease decrease back right now, your middle engaged, and your palms maintaining onto a bench for help.

3.   The leg with the foot within the loop is the running leg, so hold this thigh on the seat at some point of the motion.

four.   Initiate the motion thru slowly lifting the operating leg and straightening the knee towards the band resistance.

5.   Keep your lower leg comfortable as you enlarge your knee. Fully straighten the knee if in a function and flex your ankle.

6.   Hold an prolonged feature in quick before slowly bending the knee to move again to the begin function in a controlled motion.

7.   Complete 10-15 repetitions, then transfer legs and perform unmarried leg extensions on the other leg.

8.   Control the band on each extensions and cross again to artwork the quadriceps.

9.   You can add ankle weights to increase resistance.

Lateral Band Walks

Strengthens your hips and inner and outer thighs and improves stability. Follow the stairs below to do lateral band walks:

1.   Place a looped resistance band spherical your ankles or just above your knees if it's a whole lot much less difficult.

2.   Your feet need to be about hip-width aside alongside side your knees barely bent and palms at your elements.

3.   Take a step sideways, most important with one foot, pressing into the banded leg.

four.   Bring the alternative foot over to meet the lead foot, pressing into that leg's band.

five.   Continue taking facet steps, alternating the main foot with each step.

6.   Take small, managed steps, preserving your ft parallel and your hips consistent.

7.   Walk approximately 10 lateral steps in a single direction, then transfer and take 10 steps once more to in which you began out.

8.   Press your ft onto the ground with every step to interact your thighs.

9.   Start with slight band resistance and do more than one sets.

Balance and Stability Training

As you age, balance, and balance decline, developing the danger of falls and damage. Exercises hard stability can help seniors beautify stability on their feet. Resistance bands are a remarkable tool for enhancing stability and balance. Bands provide mild resistance and may be anchored for help on the identical time as appearing bodily activities in a standing characteristic. A everyday balance recurring with resistance bands can beef up your legs, beautify proprioception, and raise senior self perception in every day functioning.

When beginning, stand near a sturdy chair or wall for assist if desired. Proper footwear offers stability. Move slowly and attention on posture. Allow your muscles time to evolve in advance than growing trouble thru leveling up band resistance or lowering handhold assist. Gradually constructing up the duration of holds. Rest amongst durations. Aim to encompass balance carrying activities 2-3 instances every week. Here are some fantastic stability and balance education bodily games for seniors:

Side Leg Lifts

Targets your hip abductors and improves single-leg stability:

1.   Stand sideways to the anchored resistance band, going for walks the leg closest to the band.

2.   Maintain an upright posture with an engaged center and preserve your knees mild.

three. Keeping the repute leg slightly bent, slowly beautify the possibility leg in competition to the band at once out to the facet.

four.   Avoid leaning the torso or pelvis.

5.   Hold for two counts at the top.

6.   Lower the leg slowly with manage.

7.   Repeat 10 times each leg.

eight. Increase the problem with the useful aid of getting rid of the handhold or using a thicker band.

Standing Knee Raises

Improve leg coordination and dynamic balance:

1.   Stand collectively with your feet on a resistance band about hip-width apart for balance.

2.   Shift your weight to at least one leg, bending the knee barely.

three. Extend the other leg at once decrease again.

4.   Keeping the torso upright, slowly increase the once more knee in the route of the chest in opposition to resistance.

5.   Avoid leaning beforehand.

6.   Pause with the knee lifted for 1-2 seconds.

7.   Lower the leg below manipulate to the beginning position.

eight. Repeat 10 repetitions, then switch components.

nine. Progression: close your eyes on the equal time as appearing the motion.

Chapter 4: Full-Body Workouts

This financial ruin combines unique resistance band bodily sports into comprehensive physical activities focused on your vital muscle corporations. Also, shifting from better to decrease body carrying activities receives your coronary heart pumping for a awesome cardio workout. You'll be surprised at how a clean regular can work to your hands, again, chest, and legs.

These whole-body exercise physical activities will beautify your practical energy and flexibility for every day sports activities sports, like carrying groceries, getting up from a chair, and grabbing devices. It turns into less complicated at the same time as your complete frame works collectively. You'll regain energy, mobility, and stability.

Don't pass over this economic catastrophe that takes your band physical games up a notch for complete-frame transformation. When every muscle is powerful, you'll revel in an empowering experience of energy path thru your body.

Comprehensive Resistance Band Routines

Resistance band exercising exercises are a smooth but effective way to gather electricity, beautify mobility, and assist wholesome growing older. Bands provide light-weight resistance that is moderate on joints. A complete whole-body everyday hits the most muscle organizations for whole conditioning, promoting beneficial fitness so seniors stay energetic and impartial in each day lifestyles. Here are key resistance band physical video video games to encompass in a entire-frame normal.

Wood Chopper

The timber chopper is a outstanding entire-frame resistance band workout targeted for your shoulders, again muscle tissues, and middle. It improves rotational strength and mobility for your torso, this is crucial for every day sports activities like conducting, twisting to look over your shoulder, and stepping into and out of a car.

1.   Stand together collectively along with your toes hip-width aside for a robust support base.

2.   Softly bend your knees and preserve your chest lifted.

three. Hold a resistance band in every arms.

4.   Engage your middle thru lightly drawing your navel in toward your backbone to assist assist your once more at a few degree within the motion.

5.   Keeping your knees gentle, pull the band down and throughout your body in a diagonal reducing movement.

6.   Aim the band toward the alternative hip.

7.   Feel your shoulders and decrease returned muscles activating as you chop the band down and inside the path of.

8.   Slowly, in a controlled motion, go back the band up and within the path of your beginning hip.

9.   Repeat this dynamic decreasing movement for 10-15 reps on every element.

10.   Remember, breathe commonly, and maintain your abdominals braced at a few stage inside the workout.

eleven.   Avoid retaining your breath.

12.   Work at a controlled pace this is hard but possible.

thirteen.   Focus on the diagonal shoulder and torso rotation to get the most from this fantastic whole-frame toner.

Tricep Kickback

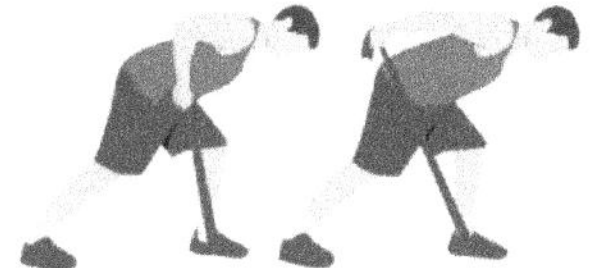

The tricep kickback is a great pass to aim the again of your higher palms and tone your tricep muscle tissues. Your triceps straighten your elbow, this is crucial for pushing motions in everyday lifestyles. This exercise will make stronger your triceps.

1.   Stand protecting one surrender of the resistance band securely below one foot to anchor it.

2.   Grasp the opposite surrender of the band within the equal-aspect hand.

3.   Keeping your pinnacle arm although, bend your elbow so your forearm lifts, bringing your hand toward your shoulder.

four.   This is your starting position.

5.   Starting from your tricep, straighten your elbow and boom your forearm proper away lower lower back within the lower back of you.

6.   Focus on squeezing your tricep muscle on the pinnacle.

7.   Hold the contraction at the pinnacle for some seconds, feeling your tricep burn.

eight. Slowly bend your elbow to go again your forearm to the start characteristic with control.

9.   Complete numerous sluggish, managed reps on one arm.

10.   Be careful no longer to jerk or swing your arm.

eleven.   Switch sides and repeat on the other arm, maintaining balance in your higher arm during.

Aim for controlled movement and precise shape. This flow will sculpt and description your triceps whilst executed frequently.

Overhead Pull-Apart

The overhead pull-aside is a top notch resistance band exercise to reinforce your pinnacle once more muscle tissues and enhance posture. Developing better lower again strength allows counteract slouching and rounding shoulders as you age.

1.   Stand keeping the resistance band taut overhead on the facet of your palms definitely extended.

2.   Engage your center muscle mass.

3.   Initiate the movement by the use of pulling your fingers outward to the perimeters in an arcing movement, squeezing your shoulder blades collectively.

4.   Hold the contraction for some seconds at the height, focusing on squeezing your top

again muscle agencies the numerous shoulder blades.

five.   Slowly bypass lower again your fingers to the beginning function overhead.

6.   Complete numerous controlled reps, being cautious now not to jerk the movement.

7.   Maintain engagement in your center muscle agencies sooner or later of to prevent excessive arching for your lower again as you pull your arms aside.

eight. Breathe normally and stand tall.

Pull-Apart

The pull-apart is a exceptional pass for strengthening your glutes and outer thighs. Your gluteal muscle groups are the primary powerhouse of your hips and butt. This exercising desires them and your hip abductors on the outer thighs for advanced hip strength.

1.   Begin the exercising thru pushing your knees outward closer to the resistance band at the identical time as squeezing your glutes.

2.   Stand together together with your feet hip-width aside.

3.   Have the resistance band looped round your thighs honestly above your knees.

four.   Concentrate on tightening your butt.

5.   Hold the peak contraction for some seconds at the same time as keeping the band taut.

6.   Your outer thighs ought to additionally enjoy this.

7.   Slowly unwind your knees to get decrease returned to the begin posture.

8.   Carry out more than one managed repetitions, taking care no longer to slouch or hip-hinge in advance.

nine.   Maintain a robust and upright torso.

10.   Throughout the overall performance, breathe commonly.

Bent-Over Row

The bent-over row is an powerful resistance band exercise for strengthening the muscles along your middle lower again. Developing muscular staying energy in your mid-lower back improves posture and permits counteract rounding shoulders.

1.   Stand maintaining the band in both hands collectively collectively with your knees barely bent.

2.   Hinge in advance at your hips to a 45-degree mindset, preserving your all over again flat.

3.   This is the starting function.

four.   Start the row with the beneficial aid of appealing your mid-again muscles.

five.   Keeping your center braced, row your elbows decrease once more, squeezing your shoulder blades.

6.   Hold the height contraction for some seconds, feeling your mid-decrease once more muscle tissues set off a number of the shoulder blades.

7.   Straighten your arms with manage to move lower again to the beginning position.

8.   Complete numerous controlled reps, being cautious not to jerk the movement.

9.   Maintain a flat once more at some stage in.

10.   Focus on squeezing your shoulder blades in vicinity of pulling together along with your palms.

11.   Breathe commonly and keep your neck snug.

Bicep Curl

The bicep curl straight away goals your biceps muscle groups at the front of your top arms. Developing sturdy biceps assists with lifting and wearing gadgets and obligations like starting jars. This pass isolates the biceps.

1.	Stand focused at the resistance band with your ft hip-width apart for balance.

2.	Hold a cope with in every hand.

3.	Let your fingers hold down at your aspects and fingers handling ahead.

four.	This is the beginning function.

five.	To start the curl, bend your elbows and curl your palms inward toward your shoulders.

6.	As you curl up, progressively agreement your biceps.

7.	Hold the contraction for a few seconds at the top.

eight.	Straighten your arms with manage to lower the handles to the begin characteristic.

nine.	Complete numerous managed reps without excessively swinging your hands.

10.	Keep your elbows near your aspects and breathe commonly within the direction of the set.

Overhead Press

The overhead press is an notable resistance band exercising for strengthening your shoulders and pinnacle another time. It works your deltoids, traps, and triceps for a toned top body definition.

1.   Stand focused on the resistance band collectively together with your ft hip-width apart for stability.

2.   Grasp a cope with in every hand.

three. Raise your palms right away overhead until your elbows are certainly extended.

four.   This is the beginning function.

5.   Start the press by using the use of attractive your shoulders and back muscle mass to press the handles immediately overhead.

6.   Hold the contraction on the pinnacle for some seconds, squeezing your shoulders.

7.   Bend your elbows with manipulate to lower the handles inside the the front of your chest.

eight. Complete numerous controlled reps, being careful now not to arch your lower decrease decrease lower back as you press up.

nine. Keep your middle muscular tissues engaged.

10.   Breathe generally and maintain your neck comfortable as you press overhead.

Front Raise

The the the front enhance is an workout on your shoulders and pinnacle lower back muscle tissues.

1.   Stand upright collectively along with your toes hip-width aside inside the center of the resistance band.

2.   While retaining your arms straight away, raise them to shoulder peak inside the the front of your body.

3. Control completely and slowly decorate your palms.

4. Hold the placement together collectively along with your arms at shoulder diploma for a count number of seconds whilst tightening your shoulder muscle groups on the top.

five. Then, gently and intentionally circulate again your palms to the start function.

6. Avoid swinging your palms fast.

7. Repeat this movement, specializing inside the use of actual shape with out swaying your torso or leaning backward as you improve your palms.

eight. Keep your middle engaged in the route of the motion.

9. Keep your shoulders cushty and keep away from shrugging or hunching them near your ears as you increase your fingers.

Banded Clams

Banded clams art work your outer hips and glutes for better balance:

1.   Start via the use of lying certainly for your issue with every knees bent at 90-degree angles.

2.   Place the resistance band snugly around your knees.

3.   Make excellent your hips are stacked and your center is engaged.

4.   Keeping both ft pressed together, slowly growth your pinnacle knee upward at the same time as rotating your hip to open the knee out to the issue.

five. Focus on maintaining your pelvis although as you raise and rotate your knee.

6.   Once your knee reaches the pinnacle of the motion, maintain this role for a few seconds.

7.   Concentrate on feeling your outer hip and glute muscle organizations have interaction as they preserve this function.

8.   Slowly lower your knee with control to return to the begin position.

9.   Be cautious now not to allow your knee drop swiftly.

10.   Complete a few managed reps on one facet, then cautiously roll over and repeat at the opportunity aspect.

11.   Try no longer to rock or twist your torso as you open and near your knees.

Banded Marching Bridge

The banded marching bridge objectives your glutes and strengthens your hips:

1.   Start via lying face up on the ground along side your knees bent at ninety degrees.

2.   Place the resistance band securely around your knees.

3.   Engage your middle muscular tissues.

4.   Keeping your neck relaxed and chin tucked, push via your heels to enhance your hips right right into a bridge position.

five.   Focus on contracting your glutes as you achieve the top.

6.   Once within the bridge, supply one knee higher toward your chest as the alternative leg presses outward closer to the band.

7.   Keep your raised knee over your hip.

8.   Hold this option for some seconds, feeling your glute and hip muscle companies running.

9.   Lower your hips to the floor and transfer knees.

10.   Continue to trade knees.

11.   Complete severa controlled reps on each thing, keeping your middle braced inside the path of the movement.

12.   Don't allow your hips sag.

Chapter 5: Customizing Your Workouts

So an extended way, the book has covered a extensive type of great resistance band physical video games. This bankruptcy shows you a way to placed all of it together into custom designed exercising routines to suit your health degree and dreams.

First, this economic disaster explores a manner to comply the physical video video games on your individual goals. Depending to your abilities, it'll offer exchange options to make movements a lot less tough or greater difficult. You need the proper resistance diploma to improvement efficiently.

The economic disaster discusses progressions and versions to keep your exercise routines powerful. As you get more potent, you may discover the way to boom to extra hard band tensions and sports activities.

With the customised hints on this economic break, you can create resistance band workout routines targeted in your problem regions and preserving you enhancing typically.

Adapting Exercises to Your Needs

Resistance bands are a awesome exercising desire for seniors because of the reality they adapt to your energy and mobility tiers. But with all this versatility comes the assignment of identifying a manner to tailor band workout physical activities effectively to satisfy your unique needs and competencies. The fantastic records is there are various techniques to regulate band physical video games to reason them to extra doable and cushty in your body. This segment discusses adapting bodily activities for your needs.

Choosing Appropriate Resistance Levels

The brilliant advantage of resistance bands is you may effortlessly regulate the intensity to suit your electricity and health. Follow these guidelines:

Start with Lighter Resistance: Begin with large, lighter bands that provide much less anxiety to permit your muscle groups time to adapt to energy education.

Focus on Form: Proper workout approach is extra crucial than how a incredible deal resistance you use. Keep correct alignment and control all through the actions.

Increase Resistance Gradually: Only waft straight away to smaller, thicker bands even as wearing sports activities turn out to be much less complex the use of lighter bands. Build up depth slowly.

Listen to Your Body: Opt for a lot a good deal less resistance if a band causes pain or is tough to preserve form. Don't rush improvement.

Adjust Band Stretch: Vary how plenty you stretch a band to make bodily sports greater hard or less difficult within the course of workout workouts. More stretch equals greater anxiety.

Use Multiple Bands: Stack bands on ankles or wrists to boom resistance as quickly as acquainted with training incrementally.

Create Asymmetry: Hold splendid resistance bands in each hand to artwork muscle groups unevenly and growth the undertaking.

Build Over Time: Proper energy education is prepared consistency through the years. Be affected individual and preserve progressing band resistance steadily as your health improves.

The key's deciding on the proper band, permitting you to keep proper approach and supplying your muscle tissues good enough resistance to growth energy over the years.

Modifying Exercises for Comfort and Safety

Listening in your body and editing the physical video games so they'll be greater snug and more secure is important whilst workout with resistance bands. Don't be afraid to make changes. Here are a few beneficial guidelines:

Play round collectively at the side of your foot positioning in the course of status sporting occasions, widening or narrowing your stance until you find out what makes balancing best. Turning your ft out barely or bringing your feet closer together can assist regular your body.

If you can't whole the complete style of movement with relevant shape, there's no disgrace in improving the exercising thru the usage of appearing partial reps indoors a controllable smaller range. Even small actions are appropriate for you.

For difficult status bodily sports that throw off your stability, preserve onto a sturdy chair, wall, or countertop for aid. It reduces the strain on muscle groups and joints for safety. There's no shame in retaining on.

Slow down and awareness on manage, jogging one limb at a time to manipulate the resistance band anxiety better. Don't do brief, jerky moves that would strain muscle agencies.

During every workout, continuously have interaction your middle muscle companies, drawing on your decrease abdominals. Activating your abs provides critical spine manual and balance for greater consistent, extra powerful workouts.

Adapting Band Workouts to Fitness Goals

Bands are useful for added than energy education. You can tailor your bodily video games to attention on precise fitness goals:

For Cardio Endurance

Resistance bands are a surely bendy exercising tool to target greater than power training. You can get innovative and tailor your band sporting activities to cognizance on enhancing one in every of a type elements of your health, like cardiovascular staying power.

If you purpose to boom your coronary coronary heart fee and beautify aerobic conditioning, your band exercise workouts can assist. Some splendid techniques to weave more heart-pumping aerobic into your resistance band intervals encompass:

Performing the strength bodily sports activities barely quicker with less rest amongst gadgets and circuits. Maintain top shape, quicken the tempo, and flow into rhythmically and constantly to raise your coronary coronary coronary heart price.

Incorporating greater physical video games associated with big overall frame actions, like squat jacks, immoderate knee runs, jumping jacks, and burpees. These dynamic multi-joint physical games spike your coronary coronary heart price.

Adding devoted aerobic-focused band wearing activities like lateral shuffle steps, speed skaters, opposite lunges with knee drives, and plyometric jumps. The band adds more resistance to make the ones cardio moves greater difficult.

Creating flowing, non-save you band workout circuits that transition seamlessly from one movement to the subsequent to keep your coronary heart price prolonged. Minimize relaxation durations.

For Improving Flexibility

Use resistance bands for the duration of stretching exercises for moderate assist and assist. The elastic band lets in you to sink deeper into stretches correctly even as engaging the targeted muscle businesses. Start with moderate resistance and popularity on slowly easing into the stretch in preference to compelling your body.

Stretch the primary muscle corporations and joints for entire flexibility. Dedicate time to seated and status stretches that open the hips, hamstrings, chest muscle tissue, shoulders, better and decrease lower returned regions, and middle stomach muscular tissues.

Concentrate on moving thru a complete form of motion on the equal time as stretching at the same time as flexing the muscle tissue being stretched. For instance, at some point of a seated hamstring stretch, have interaction the once more of the thigh with the resource of flexing the foot at the same time as leaning ahead from the hips to increase the feeling.

Hold stretches for at the least 30 seconds or longer to provide the muscular tissues time to release anxiety and elongate. Remember, breathe little by little as you stretch, and keep away from keeping your breath, that would restrict flexibility.

For Improving Balance and Stability

Single-leg carrying sports like pistol squats, lunges, and thing leg lifts strain you to activate stabilizing muscular tissues whilst promoting balance. Go slowly, maintain proper form, and handiest move as little as you can control to construct decrease frame strength.

Exercises requiring middle stabilization, like overhead shoulder presses, rotational movements, and status cable rotations, assignment your balance even as education a couple of muscle companies. Start with lighter weights if desired.

Improve common balance with controlled lateral walks, monster walks, or distinct drills displacing your center of gravity. Focus on taking large steps without problem at the equal time as maintaining your middle tight. Go gradual to begin with.

Consistency and gradual improvement are key on the equal time as enhancing flexibility and balance. Be affected man or woman, glide thoughtfully, and paintings internal your limits to soundly enhance mobility, balance, and comfort all through ordinary sports.

Listening for your frame and being inclined to adapt sports to your dreams and competencies is top to staying secure and attaining the best effects from your band bodily activities. With the right adjustments, resistance bands can assist seniors at any health level gain electricity, flexibility, and balance.

Progression and Variation

Bands offer a hard workout using body weight resistance that can be effortlessly adjusted and progressed. Creating range in band exercises continues workout sporting activities appealing with out overtaxing the frame. Here are a few key techniques seniors can upload variety to their resistance band programming.

Build Strength Gradually

Building strength is a sluggish technique requiring staying electricity and consistency. Not growing resistance too brief to avoid injury or overtraining is critical whilst the use of resistance bands. Instead, take a step-thru-step technique to allow the muscular tissues to conform at each degree.

One effective technique is to boom reps with the equal band in advance than moving to the following resistance diploma. For instance, begin by means of the use of performing an exercise for 10-12 repetitions using a moderate band till you're tired. Focus on ideal form thru the whole range of movement. Once you can complete 12 high-quality reps, upload 1-2 extra repetitions with the identical resistance. Continue growing reps in small increments till you could perform 15 reps with suitable form.

Only then switch to the subsequent heavier resistance band and drop backtrack to eight-10 reps. Allow your muscle tissues to adapt to the cutting-edge undertaking by way of way of gradually along side reps in each exercise. Over a few weeks, bring together to 12-15 fantastic reps at a higher resistance. Now, you'll be ready to development to the subsequent thicker band.

This sluggish improvement using rep additions minimizes damage threat in assessment to creating large jumps in resistance too short. Small income made normally over the years purpose extra ordinary electricity improvement. Also, it offers the joints and connective tissues time to enhance because the muscle mass expand in length and abilities.

Remember, take an afternoon of relaxation amongst jogging the same muscle businesses to allow adequate recuperation and muscle rebuilding. Building electricity requires breaking down the tissues with training and then building them up even stronger. Consistency with this slow development model will assist you benefit band power at the same time as staying healthy and active.

Adjusting Volume and Frequency

To typically flow into earlier in a resistance band application, often developing your common number of workouts offers the muscle groups with an brought challenge. Volume is the extensive shape of reps finished multiplied with the useful aid of the units. For instance, 3 devices of 10 reps equate to 30 reps.

There are some effective techniques to improvement quantity. One method is to characteristic more reps earlier than failure inside the equal gadgets. If you can entire 3 sets of 10 brilliant reps, goal to growth to 3 devices of 12-15 reps over some weeks. This ramps up the workload through 5-10 more reps in line with workout.

Another technique is together with an additional set at the same time as you obtain better reps at the particular gadgets. So, if three sets of 12 reps sense possible, add a 4th set of 10-12 reps. Both techniques observe extra extent to spur persevered earnings.

Allow enough healing among commands, working the identical muscle group even as growing quantity. For example, 48-seventy hours of relaxation is right to save you overtraining. Starting with a lower education frequency of two-three days a week for big muscle groups even as beginning a software program is wise.

Listen in your body, and don't waft quicker than your functionality to get higher. Volume should be accelerated often over a mesocycle to manipulate fatigue effectively. Adjust band anxiety first in advance than including incredible amount. Find the right stability of best volume with correct sufficient healing to improvement as it ought to be lengthy-time period.

Periodization for Ongoing Progression

Periodization is a deliberate biking approach, for persistent improvement. It varies in quantity, intensity, and frequency over set periods to strain the body in unique strategies on the same time as coping with fatigue and harm chance.

With resistance bands, periodization can start with a 4-week power-constructing mesocycle the use of decrease reps and heavier band tension. This hypertrophy section targets to boom muscle length and electricity. The subsequent four weeks have to emphasize higher reps with mild resistance to build muscular persistence.

Changing the point of interest to a new education emphasis each four-6 weeks provides a glowing stimulus in advance than variation takes place. The muscles should art work in new tactics in preference to ultimate static. These mesocycles can emerge as grade by grade more tough over a macrocycle lasting 6 months or longer.

Periodization requires strategic manipulation of education variables. For instance, developing quantity with the useful resource of together with units or reps for numerous weeks, then reducing volume however increasing intensity with the useful resource of progressing band resistance at the start of the following mesocycle. Adding rest days or restoration weeks periodically allows the frame to recharge.

Thoughtful software layout the use of periodized schooling necessities gives included development for seniors over the long term. It prevents plateaus thru planned durations of version. Working carefully with a health professional to manual band exercise choice and programming maximizes sustainable effects.

Incorporating Challenging Exercises

While frequently overloading muscle mass using heavier band resistance is powerful, consisting of multi-joint sports activities activities difficult stability and coordination is fundamental to constructing beneficial fitness. These compound movements recruit a couple of huge muscle organizations concurrently.

Exercises like squats, lunges, deadlifts, push-ups, pull-ups, and rows force you to control and stabilize your frame whilst dynamically attractive your core. It improves mobility, posture, and harm resilience for daily existence.

Start through mastering easy motion patterns like squats, hinges, and presses the usage of every legs and arms. Get cushty with the style of movement and muscle activation required. Then, try extra tough physical activities.

For instance, studying two-leg squats first gives you a basis in advance than attempting pistol squats on one leg, which requires more balance, flexibility, and electricity. Or work as a bargain as a popular push-up earlier than attempting a suspended version with increased instability.

The splendor of resistance bands is they provide lodging on the pinnacle of the motion as you arise or push away, supporting harder progressions. Bands add hassle at the go back as you lower down or pull once more.

Thoughtfully collectively with new difficult sports at the side of your modern-day exercises will ruin plateaus and construct right practical health. However, you want to progress at your tempo, studying the fundamentals earlier than trying extra complicated movements. Quality first, then amount.

Chapter 6: Advanced Techniques

In this chapter, you check superior techniques to take your exercise routines to the following degree.

First, the financial ruin explores ways to crank up your band education durations' depth to build large power and staying energy. You'll learn how to do excessive-depth c programming language education with bands to growth your coronary heart fee and fire up your muscle tissues.

Next, it covers the way to apply resistance band accessories like handles, loops, and anchors. These gear provide you with extra exercising alternatives and add challenges with the resource of centered on particular muscular tissues and motions extra precisely.

Afterward, it explains superior band sports activities activities requiring you to be greater coordinated, balanced, and on top of things. Nailing the ones dynamic actions will growth your practical health notably.

By the forestall of this monetary spoil, you'll have an high-quality toolkit of superior strategies to take your resistance schooling to the following level.

Intensifying Your Workouts

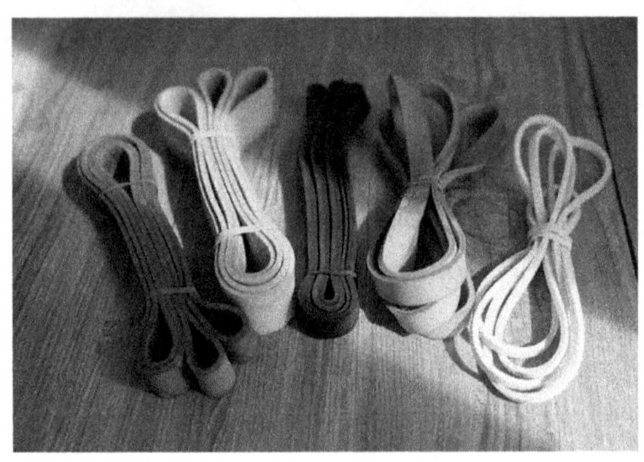

Emphasizing Eccentric and Concentric Control

Tempo and time below anxiety are the important thing variables to heighten resistance workout without usually developing the out of doors load. Moving deliberately with control emphasizes the paintings muscular tissues ought to carry out.

On the reducing or eccentric phase, consider out 3-5 seconds as you boom a muscle via its complete type of motion. Allowing gravity to boom the tissues slowly forces the muscle companies to fireside in a controlled way. For instance, slowly decrease down proper right into a whole squat in place of drop fast.

Conversely, carry or shorten muscle groups explosively on the concentric phase even as the real muscle contraction takes area. By the usage of bands, this explosive style takes benefit of the elastic draw back, helping increase you lower back up through a sticking issue. But you want to hold balance and alignment all through short lifting.

Also, pause for 1-2 seconds at any exercise's top reduced in size position or backside stretched characteristic. These isometric pauses pressure the target muscles to art work extra to stabilize and resource the body in prone joint positions.

Regardless of the fee, tempo, or time beneath load, maintain right workout shape and breathing. Rushing repetitions to keep time undermines the advantages. Extending time in each section permits fatigue muscle groups with out together with outside resistance.

Incorporating Unilateral and Multi-Planar Movements

Unilateral moves like lunges, one-arm rows, and single-leg deadlifts strain you to stabilize via the center on the same time as strolling one element at a time. It builds coordination at the same time as getting rid of power imbalances amongst components.

Since single arm and leg actions challenge stability, use lighter resistance first of all to grasp form. The unilateral load regularly feels more than bilateral versions for the reason that weight is not break up over limbs. Move slowly with manage.

Exercises concerning diagonal, transverse, and frontal aircraft actions are greater beneficial for ordinary lifestyles than sagittal aircraft physical sports like squats and presses. Chopping, lifting, and pushing in notable angles engages greater muscle fibers uniquely.

Rotational actions like Russian twists, Paloff presses, and cable chops assemble anti-rotation competencies, enhancing backbone fitness. The middle need to stand up to momentum in all guidelines. Start with low resistance, specializing in mechanics.

Placing the body underneath numerous stresses enhances mobility, balance, electricity, and strength in techniques vital again-and-forth lifts like curls or extensions cannot. But you need to draw near right shape and manipulate before trying uncommon multi-planar moves under load. Progress slowly however maintain difficult the frame.

Elevating Heart Rate with Reduced Rest Periods

Shortening rest intervals spikes the coronary coronary heart charge and popular workout intensity efficaciously. Limiting downtime amongst devices and physical video games forces you to paintings greater tough as fatigue accumulates.

Reducing relaxation to 30-45 seconds between gadgets restricts how an lousy lot the muscular tissues can recover earlier than exercise them another time. Also, it'll boom desires on the cardiovascular tool to deliver oxygen and clean metabolic waste.

Move fluidly amongst sports sports, centered on specific body additives to hold your pulse accelerated. For example, go with the flow from squats to push-u.S.A.To rows with out extra rest. Keep actual artwork time high and relaxation periods quick and active.

Maintaining consistent motion with minimal prolonged sitting or reputation maximizes calorie burn at some stage in the session. The cumulative fatigue forces your coronary heart to pump at higher fees to gas walking muscles.

This greater appropriate metabolic conditioning offers cardiovascular blessings while burning greater body fat. Use suitable resistance. Your shape and method must not fail due to fatigue. Monitor your attempt stages and preserve rest intervals short however enough.

The greater active time instead of relaxation time in the path of a band exercise, the more the functionality advantages. But don't beneath-get higher amongst intense devices, otherwise you undermine electricity income. Find the most perfect stability.

Advanced Exercise Progressions and Techniques

Continue advancing carrying events into extra tough versions or the usage of device presenting instability to save you plateaus. After mastering conventional physical sports, try unilateral versions like cut up squats in place of regular squats or unmarried-arm chest presses over dual palms.

The decreased balance works the middle and ancillary stabilizers masses greater to keep form and balance. If less complicated variations enjoy snug, shifting to the ones unmarried limb or repute sports activities marks an development and milestone in your health tiers.

Also, incorporate device like workout balls, suspension walking footwear, or gliding discs into your physical games. Performing presses, rows, or squats with these devices will increase the stability and control required than robust surfaces. The muscle tissue music in to maintain posture.

Trying new bodily video games forcing the frame to move unfamiliarly complements neuromuscular activation and knowledge improvement. Movements like landmine presses, pull-overs, and rotational lifts pressure muscle tissues in a unique way.

Learning new techniques guarantees you in no way get the identical stimulus for too lengthy. However, you want to apprehend form at decrease intensities in advance than adding resistance bands. Don't development too quick beyond your capability.

Variety is essential for lengthy-time period version and talents building. Progressing exercise choice, gear, and versions provide integrated techniques to heighten band physical activities. Remember, improvement step by step at your pace.

Incorporating Challenging Metabolic Circuits

Metabolic resistance training circuits are a time-green manner to maximize fat burning and conditioning with bands. These excessive-depth circuits transition seamlessly among sports, centered on wonderful motion styles and muscle groups with minimum rest.

Combine four-6 body physical sports proper into a flowing circuit, which include push-ups, rows, contrary lunges, rotations, and band pull-aparts. Perform them consecutively with 15-30 seconds of rest between actions to keep the coronary coronary coronary heart price prolonged.

Sequence complimentary carrying sports permit certain muscle companies to in quick get higher at the identical time as others are worked. For example, follow an pinnacle push workout with a decrease pull bypass. Then, transition to center or single leg paintings earlier than returning to the top body.

Moving rhythmically between bodily sports annoying situations the muscular and cardiovascular structures concurrently. Repeat the whole circuit 2-four instances in step with your health and decided on depth.

Always pick out appropriate resistance. Some fatigue is ideal sufficient, however the form shouldn't in reality harm down. Maintain proper pacing so that you paintings difficult however live on pinnacle of things. Proper method prevents harm.

With minimum time invested, the ones dynamic metabolic circuits offer a thorough exercising in one exercise bout. They maximize energy expenditure for weight loss on the same time as enhancing muscular and cardiovascular staying strength.

Monitoring Intensity through Perceived Exertion

Rather than relying on random out of doors metrics, pay attention to your body's cues to gauge exercise depth because it ought to be. Rate your perceived exertion on a 1-10 scale, with 1 being rest and 10 being exhaustion.

Aim for tough however sustainable intensity, ideally 6 to eight on the scale for max resistance band workouts. The weight or resistance ought to sense pretty tough with the aid of manner of the final focused reps however no longer not viable to complete with right shape.

The "speak take a look at" is also a useful depth manual. You need to speak coherently via physical sports but aren't able to certainly sing, which requires extra oxygen. The depth is actually too excessive in case you can't say a few phrases without gasping heavily.

Detecting whilst muscle mass begin tiring, respiration turns into more rapid, and also you harm a slight sweat are more crucial signs and symptoms and signs than hitting high first-class coronary heart charge zones, speeds, or strength outputs. Your subjective perceived attempt helps optimize the stimulus while minimizing harm danger.

Of path, preserve the intensity inside a while-commemorated fitness desires and capabilities. In c programming language training, aggressive athletes and further conditioned human beings can preserve higher exertion stages than elegant populace exercising routines. Intensity need to be in my opinion appropriate.

Chapter 7: Staying Safe and Injury-Free

At this aspect to your resistance band training, retaining healthful and heading off accidents is fundamental to progressing. This bankruptcy devices out recommendations to help you work out very well and keep your health prolonged-term.

First, the bankruptcy covers common mistakes to persuade clean of while using resistance bands, like bad shape, overtraining, and incorrectly the usage of the bands. Learning to repair the ones errors will let you maintain training correctly.

The economic ruin moreover explores proactive guidelines for looking after your joints and muscles as you growth. The aim is to provide you the statistics to live damage-loose and get the most out of your physical games. You've already positioned inside the hard artwork. So, this bankruptcy guarantees you could hold resistance schooling successfully. By the give up of this monetary disaster, you'll assemble resilience and hold the fitness profits you've worked so tough for.

Common Mistakes to Avoid

Resistance bands deliver seniors clean, effective techniques to strength teach at home. The elastic bands provide moderate to heavy resistance ranges the use of easy body weight exercises. Resistance schooling offers large advantages for seniors, which includes increased electricity, mobility, bone density, and fall prevention even as used nicely.

However, there are a few common errors seniors must keep away from at the same time as appearing resistance band exercising sports. Improper shape, an excessive amount of resistance, bad anchoring, and insufficient heat-u.S.A. Of americacan undermine effects and cause harm. Being privy to the ones capacity mistakes allows seniors maximize the blessings of resistance band carrying sports at the equal time as exercising efficiently.

1.	Choosing Bands with Too Much Resistance

When starting a resistance band program, many ambitious seniors make the error of choosing bands with resistance ranges which might be too difficult. Elastic resistance bands are available in a large style of intensities, from very mild to noticeably heavy resistance. Grabbing the most rugged, hardcore-searching band from the start is tempting. However, seniors need to choose out lighter, beginner bands after they first embark on resistance schooling.

Advanced heavy resistance bands can strain growing antique muscle businesses and joints, fundamental to harm if used in advance. Starting with an excessive amount of resistance frequently reasons seniors to compensate thru the use of terrible form and momentum to complete reps. This mistake undermines effectiveness and imprints risky movement styles. Even seniors who are lively and conditioned in cardiovascular exercising need to start resistance schooling with mild bands.

Mastering superb form and technique on the equal time as building your energy foundation takes precedence over intensity at the same time as beginning. Light and mild resistance bands permit seniors to do that at the same time as maintaining manage and balance. Seniors would likely enjoy self-aware, starting with very mild, "wimpy" looking crimson and yellow bands. But those teach safe handling and movements to improvement from.

Attempting advanced wearing sports like lunges or presses with heavy bands too fast risks torn muscle groups or broken tendons. If the band suddenly pulls seniors out of alignment, it is possibly to be tough. Progress up the resistance ranges incrementally after organising competence and electricity. Seniors in a rush to heighten resistance hazard ache and damage, so be conservative and affected character at the same time as selecting initial bands.

2.	Insufficient Warm-Ups

Many senior exercisers eager to start their resistance band physical games make the mistake of no longer warming up properly in advance. A right warmness-up is crucial schooling in advance than any electricity education routine.

Dynamic warmness-united stateslasting as a minimum five-10 mins must come to be famous for seniors earlier than using resistance bands. Light cardiovascular interest will boom blood flow to the muscles. Moving joints fluidly through whole ranges of motion, like elbow and knee bends, lubricates joints and enhances mobility. Also, the usage of slight resistance bands or tubes gently turns on muscle agencies.

Warm-up devices of intended carrying activities with minimal resistance assist top the neuromuscular device. Higher rep gadgets of 10-15 with less tough resistance bands essentially trick the body and thoughts into looking in advance to hobby. It ramps up recognition and alignment earlier than heavier gadgets. Insufficient heat-u.S.A.Cause tighter muscle corporations, confined variety of motion, and compromised power.

Properly warming up loosens connective tissues, elevates coronary heart charge and body temperature, and mentally prepares seniors for education disturbing situations in advance. Explosive power and muscle stamina boom in comparison to cold starts offevolved with out dynamic heat-ups. Insufficient warmth-u.S.A.Raise harm dangers like strained muscles from stunning the frame with surprising resistance. Consistent dynamic heat-usaimprove typical performance and safety.

3.   Poor Exercise Form

Many seniors workout with resistance bands make the error of prioritizing dreams like velocity, reps, and circuits over proper form. Form frequently suffers in the quest to keep up immoderate pacing or complete immoderate volumes. However, the right method and alignment want to generally take priority with resistance training.

Band resistance applies delivered pressure all through joints and muscle corporations. The horrible form gets amplified into feasible traces or tears. Common form errors like immoderate lower again arching, jutting the pinnacle ahead, or twisting shoulders dangerously have to be prevented.

Controlled, specific motions are key, even though they entire fewer reps. Bracing abdominals, keeping actions aligned, and refraining from using momentum all enhance your effects and guard getting old joints. Rushing through reps without regard for form frequently ends in harm.

Resistance bands allow effective modifications to be shape-terrific for seniors with barriers. But compromising foundational posture concepts is unwise. Spinal health have to be supported via impartial neck, midback, and pelvis positioning.

four.   Not Engaging Core Muscles

Many seniors do not truely engage their center stabilizer muscle corporations even as performing resistance band physical video video games. It reduces potential blessings and might lead to lower returned strain over time. Making middle activation a concern with band education enhances consequences and spinal protection.

The middle muscle companies offer crucial spine stabilization in the route of repute sporting sports activities like squats, presses, and rows. Poor center recruitment in the route of band workout routines stresses the again for the purpose that bands pull joints out of steady positioning without engaged abdominals.

Consciously pull your navel towards your backbone to artwork the deep center muscle companies. Cues like "zip up your middle" let you do not forget to fire those postural muscle corporations. Activated glute muscle mass hold pelvic neutrality for lower again fitness, and maintaining your shoulders extensive and down engages scapular stabilizers.

Rigorously bracing the core transfers power from massive muscle groups to the bands extra efficaciously. Active cores help you balance at some point of unilateral or standing movements. Make appealing the middle a concern in advance than appearing reps.

5.   Inadequate Anchoring of Bands

Many seniors exercise with resistance bands anchored to furnishings or doors in their homes. These makeshift anchors are often risky and loosen sooner or later of exercising exercises, and bands snap lower decrease returned unexpectedly inside the route of clients. Investing in a dedicated resistance band anchor device significantly enhances safety.

Reliance on anchors like near doors, table legs, or carabiners often fail. Anchors turn out to be dislodged, bands slip via cracks, or friction offers way through repeated use. A sudden release of resistance bands can reason seniors to lose balance, increasing falls. Unsecured bands will snap again forcefully, raising damage dangers.

High-great portable door anchors the usage of reinforced straps boom protection for anchoring your bands. Some systems have twin anchor factors on each side of the band to provide stability via the whole sort of movement. Advanced anchors with swivel connections deliver introduced safety if the character loses grip at the bands mid-exercising.

Properly anchoring resistance bands maintains seniors more secure whilst letting them maximize workout benefits. Secure anchors provide regular resistance for fuller muscle activation, so have a examine options to discover anchors with clean installation but organisation-grade durability. Protect protection and decorate home resistance schooling with robust band anchors.

6.   Overarching Bands

Many seniors mistake looping heavy resistance bands truly over the tops in their ft or shoulders even as workout. However, this constricts float and must be averted. Overarching bands can numb arms and feet and bring about bad exercise mechanics.

Bands wrapped genuinely over your foot or shoulders press tightly into the tendons with repeated motions. This reduces blood go along with the drift, causing tingling or numbness within the ft or hands. Overarching bands furthermore restriction the shape of motion by way of using stopping joints from moving via whole extensions and contractions.

Instead, seniors need to anchor bands securely beneath the midfoot for decrease frame sporting occasions. Padded ankle straps are each exclusive choice that disperses pressure. Handles and cuffs lightly distribute anxiety for higher frame movement, stopping constriction and allowing fuller motion.

Pay near interest to symptoms and signs and symptoms like tingling, numbness, or "falling asleep" of extremities even as the use of resistance bands. These signs and signs sign constriction requiring right now adjustment. Avoid truely wrapping bands over joints the least bit fees.

7.   Holding Breath

Many seniors inadvertently keep their breath whilst exerting in the route of resistance bands. However, this can dangerously spike blood pressure and need to be averted. Remember, breathe continuously, even in some unspecified time in the future of hard repetitions.

Holding your breath frequently takes location while you're doing hard reps and bracing extra hard in opposition to resistance. However, this motives blood stress to upward thrust unsafely because the coronary heart struggles to pump within the direction of closed airlines. Make a concerted effort to exhale for the duration of the exertion phase and inhale on the pass lower lower back.

If you cannot breathe without difficulty inside the path of the motion, the resistance degree is just too immoderate. Continuing devices at the same time as retaining breath locations excessive pressure on the coronary heart. Seniors with pre-present cardiac or blood pressure troubles ought to be mainly cautious.

Keep reps controlled and breathe rhythmically even if the band resistance intensifies. Avoid maintaining your breath to the detail of dizziness or lightheadedness. Resistance schooling need to no longer enjoy like every-out sprinting. You want to count on harder respiratory, but avoid holding your breath.

eight. Insufficient Recovery amongst Workouts

Many bold seniors make the error of overtraining through not allowing enough healing time among resistance band intervals. However, true enough recuperation is important for muscle electricity enhancements. Avoid exercising the equal muscular tissues on decrease back-to-lower once more days.

Overtraining hinders outcomes via not giving muscle tissues the vital rest to regenerate and adapt. Optimizing electricity income calls for a stability of stressing muscle tissues and permitting healing. Work unique predominant muscle groups each consultation and take at least one complete relaxation day each week.

Schedule top body, lower frame, and center carrying sports activities over excellent durations spaced aside. Allowing more than one days earlier than repeating the same muscle businesses prevents overuse. Also, adjust volume and intensity if pain persists for more than one days in a while.

Seniors construct electricity and muscle sooner or later of relaxation days even as workout. Recovery permits protein synthesis and muscle rebuilding to occur. Resistance education with insufficient healing amongst sporting events leads to frustration and plateaus, so be affected man or woman and guide education with proper rest.

Managing Joint and Muscle Health

It is important that seniors well control joint and muscle health even as appearing the ones exercising routines to keep away from harm. Here's an in-depth have a look at of joint and muscle health troubles for seniors doing resistance band sports activities sports.

Understanding Age-Related Changes

As you age, your muscle tissue and joints undergo natural and inevitable modifications, making exercising greater tough and precarious. Muscle mass and muscular electricity decrease drastically, specially after human beings attain 50 years antique.

The joints within the frame are inclined to emerge as stiffer and masses less flexible, with extra put on and tear from many years of use. As seniors age, those modifications and changes suggest older adults need to modify and modify their exercise applications to cope with their decreased competencies.

Proper changes and modifications to workout routines are critical to account for decreased muscle groups and joint flexibility. If not adjusted for the ones age-associated bodily modifications, exercising programs can come to be volatile via the usage of manner of overexerting the muscle agencies and joints.

Muscle Changes

Muscles reduce lower back in duration and kind of fibers with developing older. This loss of muscle businesses is called sarcopenia. Less muscle way much less strength to perform every day sports. Also, muscular tissues come to be an awful lot a good deal less inexperienced at generating energy for motion. These factors growth the risk of falls and accidents.

Joint Changes

Cartilage, the clean, slippery tissue protective and protecting the joints' surfaces, regularly wears down and deteriorates with age. This age-related breakdown of cartilage reasons joint stiffness, achiness, pain, and reduced flexibility and kind of movement.

Inflammation in the joint areas will increase with senior years, compounding and exacerbating joint signs and symptoms and symptoms. Seniors' joints have reduced functionality to soak up the shocks and impact of exercise and regular actions. Therefore, older joints are greater liable to injuries, along with strains, sprains, tears, and elegant overuse from physical interest.

Deterioration of joint cartilage and prolonged irritation lessen the joint's inborn resilience and predispose seniors to painful joint injuries. Seniors should be aware about joint ache alerts, employ right shape, drift via complete degrees of movement, and allow for proper enough rest and recuperation among exercising intervals to keep away from harm. Protecting joint health improves the excellent of existence for seniors.

To account for age-associated physical changes, resistance band exercises are best low-impact bodily video games:

1.   Start with Low Resistance

Heavier resistance overloads muscle businesses and joints. Beginners need to begin with lighter resistance bands and enhance cautiously. Never workout thru joint pain.

2.   Focus on the Full Range of Motion

Avoid positions that overly compress or torque joints. Move through a cushty kind of motion, retaining manipulate. A entire sort of movement promotes mobility.

3.   Use Proper Form and Alignment

Correct form reduces damage threat and ensures muscle agencies are worked efficiently. Keep a unbiased backbone function with the aid of way of attractive center muscle mass. Move slowly. Don't "snap" joints into role.

4.   Allow for Recovery

Aging muscle agencies want more time to recover amongst physical games, so time table relaxation days among lessons. Consider lighter resistance or shorter physical games if pain persists.

five.   Include Balance Exercises

Balance declines with age, growing falls. Exercise sporting events want to embody standing leg swings, facet steps, and toe and heel lifts. Have manual close by if wanted.

Managing Specific Joints and Muscles

Certain joints and muscle agencies deserve precise interest and interest at the same time as seniors workout with resistance bands to avoid damage.

1.   Shoulders: The shoulder joints and surrounding muscle tissues are at risk of lines and tears as you age. Seniors have to keep away from excessive overhead stretches in the course of resistance carrying occasions, that might irritate the rotator cuff muscle organizations. Always control the movement whilst executing shoulder presses, rows, and rotations.

2.   Elbows: The elbow joint and its tendons are at elevated hazard for painful infection and tendonitis from overuse with exercise bands. Keep the wrists straight away and the elbows near the frame, not flared outward, all through bicep curls and tricep extensions. Don't hyperextend your joints.

3.   Wrists: Wrists end up at risk of carpal tunnel syndrome and osteoarthritis with age. Limit immoderate bending again or twisting of the wrists during exercise. Choose a independent wrist function whilst grasping

bands, and recall using wrist braces or helps if wished.

4.   Lower Back: The lumbar backbone and lower again muscular tissues are more at risk of disc degeneration, compressed nerves, and painful muscle traces with age. Maintain neutral alignment of the decrease once more without arching or rounding. Brace the center throughout squats, deadlifts, and resisted pulls or rows.

five.   Knees: Knee joints are regularly afflicted with osteoarthritis and susceptible to ligament tears the older you get. Perform all leg sporting sports through a snug style of movement with out forcing or locking your knees right away. Avoid ache with the useful resource of no longer exceeding your flexibility limits.

6.   Ankles and Feet: These joints steadily lose everyday mobility and flexibility with senior years. Select pretty pretty a number motion and positioning for ankle and foot bodily video games that do not excessively

strain the joints. Practice seated wearing occasions to take weight off the ankles if wanted.

7.   Core Muscles: Torso center muscle groups are essential for stability, posture, decrease returned help, and balance in some unspecified time in the future of exercising and each day interest. Include core movements like planks, crunches, and side bends. Gradually growth middle strength. Don't overdo it early on.

eight. Hips: Hip joints and surrounding muscle groups want to be exercised to preserve mobility, no longer overstretched or strained. Keep your knees over your ankles in popularity moves. Avoid hip pain with the resource of restricting immoderate the front-to-once more or facet-to-facet leg motions.

9.   Chest: The pectoral muscular tissues may be efficiently strengthened with resisted chest presses. Avoid shoulder impingement with the resource of preserving your elbows beneath your shoulders and no longer

overextending the joints. Maintain a small arch within the lower again via engaging the center.

10.   Hamstrings: This susceptible muscle group at the again of the thighs is vulnerable to strains and stiffness with age. Stretch the hamstrings thoroughly. Perform hamstring curls gently without over-bending the knees. Limit resistance and type of movement to save you harm.

Chapter 8: Lifestyle and Nutrition

Your way of life selections and nutrients have a big effect on retaining your health dreams inside the long term. This financial ruin gives way of life and diet tips tailor-made for seniors to supplement your exercises.

First, the chapter affords vitamins hints targeted on fueling your workout exercises and helping regular health. You'll learn how to shape your weight-reduction plan to energise your training, construct lean muscle, and meet your frame's converting desires. The financial disaster covers key vitamins to guide bone density, joint health, and immune characteristic.

It discusses integrating fitness into your every day existence as a senior. The motive is to present you the device to maximise your high-quality of existence and capability through smart lifestyle and vitamins options. This way, you'll maintain your body acting and feeling top notch as you embody resistance training for lifelong health.

Nutrition Tips for Seniors

Proper vitamins is crucial for seniors actively electricity education with resistance bands. The right weight loss program gives strength for exercising routines, fuels muscle growth, and supports joint fitness. This phase offers nutrients guidelines tailored to senior resistance band exercisers inside the following regions:

1.   Getting Enough Protein

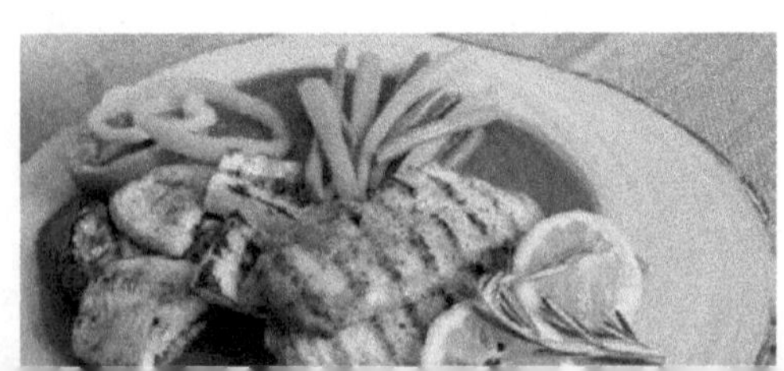

Consuming adequate protein is considerably essential for seniors doing resistance band training to assemble and restore the muscle fibers that get broken down at some point of resistance physical games. Seniors have in particular excessive protein dreams specially to combat sarcopenia, the age-associated lack of muscle tissues and energy. Without sufficient protein from your diet regime, you're liable to dropping the muscle you strive to build up.

How Much Protein?

The advocated each day protein consumption for senior resistance trainees is 0.Five-0.7 grams of protein regular with pound of body weight. For a senior who weighs a hundred fifty pounds, this equates to 75-100 grams of protein for the day. It is proper to region this protein consumption evenly inside the path of the day over important food and snacks in vicinity of ingesting it in a unmarried sitting. Spreading it out approach there is probably a ordinary deliver to the muscle groups. Due to sarcopenia, older adults need protein on the better give up of the range.

High-Quality Protein Foods

Some terrific meals property of fantastic protein consist of eggs, fowl like bird and turkey, fatty fish like salmon and tuna, Greek yogurt and other dairy products, beans, nuts collectively with almonds and walnuts, and soy meals like tofu and edamame. Supplemental protein powders made from whey and casein can also help seniors meet every day protein intake desires if they'll be having trouble ingesting enough protein-rich whole meals, that is commonplace.

Timing of Protein

Consuming protein earlier than and after resistance workout routines is likewise encouraged to supply muscle tissues. Seniors ought to purpose for 20-30 grams of protein from a meal or snack interior 30 minutes after workout to maximise muscle restore and boom. Good submit-exercising protein alternatives encompass a Greek yogurt smoothie with berries or a turkey sandwich. Pre-exercising protein is also beneficial. Aim for 20 grams about an hour earlier than resistance schooling to offer your muscle groups with amino acids during the consultation.

2.   Consuming Enough Calories

Resistance training substantially will boom seniors' normal calorie and electricity wishes. When seniors do no longer devour enough power to meet the ones multiplied wishes, the frame is pressured to interrupt down muscular tissues for fuel, defeating resistance workout's reason. To assist muscle building, seniors who are actively power schooling have to:

Increase their regular baseline calorie intake with the aid of manner of approximately 15% on the instances of resistance band workout sporting events. For example, if a senior commonly eats 1600 energy each day, intention for approximately 1840 power on exercise days.

Consume a similarly hundred-300 strength on non-workout days to account for improved muscle businesses and metabolism.

Focus on getting those greater power from nutrient-dense complete substances in preference to empty resources like soda, candy, and chips. Quality energy from wholesome fat, complex carbs, and proteins will gasoline exercising routines properly.

If you gain unwanted fat benefit, you could lower regular energy barely on the same time as retaining your protein consumption immoderate. Cutting energy too substantially leads to muscle loss, so purpose for a modest calorie growth to guide resistance schooling. Consulting with a dietitian will assist you figure out the proper amount of energy you want.

three. Staying Hydrated

Muscle tissue accommodates about 75% water, highlighting the crucial element feature of hydration in muscle fitness and function. Not eating sufficient and turning into dehydrated can extensively abate resistance schooling performance and recovery.

Daily Fluid Intake

Seniors need to drink at the least 8 cups of non-caffeinated, non-alcoholic fluids every day as a cutting-edge baseline to hold top hydration. On resistance exercise days, fluid consumption want to be advanced to 10-12 cups of water in addition to unique beverages to replace extra fluid losses from sweat.

Hydrating During Workouts

Proper hydration during schooling sessions is essential. Aim to sip about four-6 ounces. Of water each 15-20 minutes at the same time as actively exercising to constantly update fluid loss from sweat. Drink water earlier than, more than one instances in a few unspecified time within the future of, and after completing the resistance band exercising. Proper hydration will assist seniors whole greater reps.

Monitoring Hydration

Paying interest to urine color is an smooth way to gauge your every day hydration reputation. Generally, faded yellow to clear urine signs adequate hydration. Dark yellow, smelly-smelling urine generally indicates dehydration and the need to drink extra fluids. Seniors should watch for wonderful signs and symptoms and signs of dehydration like headache, cramping, dizziness, and fatigue sooner or later of exercise routines and normal lifestyles. Keeping nicely hydrated reduces damage threat and enables resistance education earnings.

4.   Vitamins and Minerals

Several key micronutrients are particularly vital for seniors engaged in resistance education to assist muscle, bone, and joint fitness.

Calcium and Vitamin D: Calcium and vitamins D are vital for retaining bone density and energy and helping muscle contractions. Good meals property include yogurt, milk, leafy greens like spinach, and fatty fish. Many seniors additionally want supplemental nutrients D3 to make sure properly enough consumption for bone and muscle health.

Vitamin C: Vitamin C aids the frame in producing collagen and cartilage to keep healthful joint surfaces. It has antioxidant houses to lessen inflammatory damage. Citrus quit result, broccoli, peppers, strawberries, and kiwi offer weight loss plan C.

Iron: Iron permits the frame to offer hemoglobin, the protein in red blood cells that includes oxygen to running muscle groups. Adequate iron prevents anemia and associated fatigue. Iron is located in pork, hen, seafood, spinach, nuts, beans, and iron-fortified whole grains.

Magnesium and Zinc: Magnesium and zinc are key in muscle contractions and protein synthesis. Excellent property encompass nuts, seeds, beans, shellfish, yogurt, fatty fish, avocado, chickpeas, oatmeal, and pumpkin seeds.

Omega-3s: The anti-inflammatory omega-three fatty acids EPA and DHA resource joint, coronary heart, and mind health. Fatty fish like salmon and sardines, walnuts, flaxseeds, and chia seeds are suitable belongings.

Consuming those nutrients and minerals via materials or super dietary supplements can offer seniors with key nutrients to help maximize resistance training benefits.

5.   Powering Workouts with Carbs

Carbohydrates are vital in fueling seniors for their resistance training durations and powering via workout routines. Senior resistance trainees generally need approximately 3-5 grams of carbohydrates constant with pound of frame weight daily to fulfill expanded electricity needs. Focusing on getting those carbs from nutrient-dense, excessive-fiber property for sustained energy is crucial.

Fruits and Vegetables: Fruits, greens, critical nutrients, minerals, fiber, and antioxidants provide carbohydrates to aid schooling. Aim for eight-10 servings each day.

Whole Grains: Whole grain belongings of carbs like oatmeal, quinoa, brown rice, entire wheat bread, and pasta deliver normal, prolonged-lasting strength and fiber to meet you. Choose one hundred% complete grains over subtle alternatives.

Starchy Vegetables: Starchy veggies, in conjunction with potatoes, candy potatoes, peas, butternut squash, carrots, and corn, are carbohydrates to fuel exercise energy. Consume lots of colorations.

Pre-Workout Carbs: Consuming a carbohydrate-containing snack 30-60 mins before resistance periods can maximize strength and performance. Good options are oatmeal with fruit, entire grain toast with avocado, or a banana with peanut butter.

Focusing on interesting, fiber-wealthy carb assets deliver seniors sustained power for resistance sessions without blood sugar spikes and crashes. Properly fueling physical games leads to greater effective schooling.

6.   Supporting Joints and Connective Tissue

The repetitive stress of resistance training can take a toll in your joint fitness. Consuming vitamins supporting joints and connective tissues can help hold joints flexible and resilient.

Collagen: Collagen is the primary structural protein in connective tissues like tendons and ligaments. Consuming collagen-wealthy bone broth or hydrolyzed collagen nutritional supplements can offer the constructing blocks to reinforce this connective tissue community and resist schooling stress.

Glucosamine and Chondroitin: Glucosamine and chondroitin are compounds that rise up manifestly in wholesome cartilage. Supplements with those vitamins can help restore and make more potent broken cartilage. Evidence is mixed, however a few discover remedy from joint ache.

Antioxidants: Colorful end cease end result and veggies, dark chocolate, inexperienced tea, and red wine embody antioxidants combating infection and unfastened radical damage to joints and tissues from resistance schooling. Berries, tart cherry juice, citrus quit result, and dark leafy vegetables are suitable assets.

Seniors need to recall awesome joint-excellent nutrients like omega-three fatty acids from fish oil, curcumin from turmeric, and avocado soybean unsaponifiables (ASU). A weight loss plan rich in natural anti-inflammatories can assist maintain seniors' joints resilient.

7.   Avoiding Counterproductive Habits

Skipping Meals: Skipping food results in large gaps in energy, vitamins, and protein consumption, inflicting the body to interrupt down muscle mass for gasoline, it's far counterproductive for building strength. Seniors need to intention to devour often, about each 3-4 hours, to preserve strength and constantly deliver muscle agencies. Eat breakfast internal an hour of waking to refuel after the in a single day rapid.

Consuming Excess Sugar: While sugar tastes particular, consuming chocolates and desserts in more can spike blood sugar and boom irritation in the body, potentially slowing down recuperation from exercising. Limit delivered sugars with the useful resource of retaining off sodas, sweet, ice cream, and baked objects. Instead, choose out smooth fruit, clean yogurt, and entire grains like oats and quinoa for carbohydrates and splendor. The nutrients and antioxidants in herbal food counter inflammation.

Restricting Calories Too Much: Cutting power too aggressively on a each day basis will reduce the energy and protein to be had for excessive resistance workout routines and can cause muscle breakdown. Mild calorie cut price of a hundred-200 power can assist seniors lose fats at the same time as keeping muscle mass. But too steep of a deficit undercuts training. Determine minimum electricity in your hobby stage and reduce slightly for fat loss.

Skipping Pre-Workout Fuel: Never do resistance education on an empty belly first factor in the morning. The lack of protein, carbs, and hydration will cause low energy, strength, and stamina inside the path of the consultation. Always have a pre-workout meal or snack with protein, carbs, and fluid at the least an hour earlier so muscular tissues have good enough fuel. A piece of fruit and protein shake is an smooth choice.

Under-Hydrating: Chronically dehydration hampers physical staying electricity and power, potentially developing joint ache and susceptibility to lines or pulls. Make hydration a each day dependancy via way of ingesting water and one-of-a-kind fluids even whilst you're no longer thirsty. Carry a water bottle as a reminder. Proper hydration energizes physical games, aids muscle recuperation, and continues joints cushioned.

Chapter 9: Success Stories

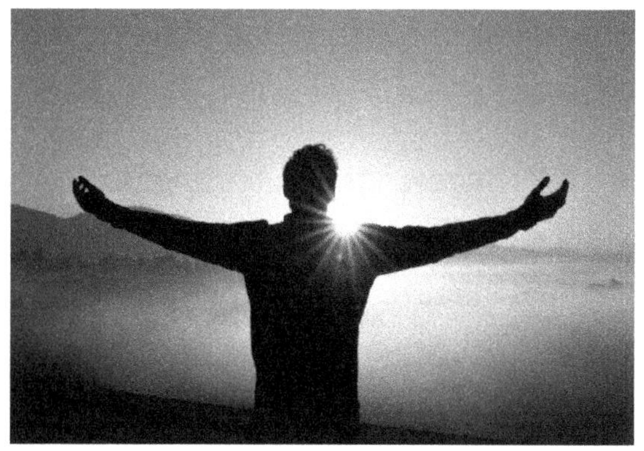

You did it. You've made it to the final bankruptcy. Throughout the book, you've long gone over the perks of resistance band education and been given numerous hints to start your health adventure. Now comes the best issue. This bankruptcy relays right memories of inspiring older adults who used bands to transform their fitness.

In this motivational financial catastrophe, you'll have a look at approximately outstanding ladies and men who overcame annoying conditions and completed essential profits thru dedicated band workouts. Despite handling troubles like damage, infection, and growing older, they made wonderful improvement in constructing power, mobility, and power.

Their bills show the uplifting energy of resistance schooling to reinforce physical and intellectual health. These seniors display off excessive grit within the face of adversity and resilience to maintain enhancing regardless.

The aim of this chapter is for their inspirational stories to encourage you to use resistance bands as a device to step up your health and abilties.

Real-Life Testimonials

Testimonial 1 (Andrew)

At age 72, Andrew turn out to be bored with feeling inclined and frail. Simple sports like hiking stairs or wearing groceries had turn out to be chores. He knew he desired a alternate to beautify his power, mobility, and independence. On his doctor's recommendation, he started the usage of resistance bands for workout exercises at home. In exceptional 2 months, he determined a dramatic distinction. His balance and stability had significantly stepped forward, and he now not felt shaky taking walks or modified into concerned approximately falling. Also, his top body felt greater muscular and toned. Activities like lifting heavy pots inside the kitchen or doing circle of relatives upkeep had been simpler now. He credited his transformation to the resistance band exercising sporting activities he did 3 times consistent with week. The bands supplied effective power schooling with out joint ache or impact. He did severa wearing occasions like bicep curls, rows, presses, and squats to goal all his essential muscle tissues. As the bands stretched over the years, he superior to higher resistance stages to usually challenge himself. His spouse changed into so inspired with the changes she commenced doing band workout routines with him. He felt a long time extra younger and had renewed fitness and power.

Resistance bands gave him his electricity and mobility lower lower back.

Testimonial 2 (Margaret)

As a seventy eight-yr-antique, Margaret had come to simply accept that aches, pains, and vulnerable component have been a part of developing older. She confined herself to mild sports activities due to the reality some thing too strenuous become too tough on her body. But on the same time as her grandkids visited one summer time, she struggled to maintain up and knew some problem needed to change. She started out the usage of resistance bands and following exercising movies created for seniors. The consequences had been lifestyles-converting. After 3 months of regular band training, getting down on the floor to play alongside side her grandkids, she no longer required help to stand back up. Her balance had advanced pretty, so she had no more issues approximately tripping or losing her footing. Gardening, cleaning, and buying have been lots much less complicated with improved leg, hip, and decrease back energy. The bands had been so bendy she targeted each muscle corporation for whole body conditioning. She felt more youthful, extra healthful, and extra colourful than she had in a long term. Using resistance bands had empowered her to be lively and maintain up collectively together with her grandkids. She only wanted she had started out strength training faster. It is by no means too past due to beautify your abilties and stay existence to the fullest.

Testimonial 3 (James)

As an active 80-year-vintage, James prided himself on being in shape for his age. That come to be till a fall led to a damaged hip and a extended recuperation. He out of place electricity and mobility and struggled to regain his in advance health. On his physical therapist's advice, he started out out education with resistance bands. The flexibility of the bands allowed him to exercising even as warding off further joint strain at some point of his healing. After only 1 month, he found crucial upgrades in his electricity, stability, and type of motion. Now, years later, bands are even though his bypass-to for staying lively and unbiased. He did upper and decrease body sporting sports like shoulder presses, bicep curls, squats, and kickbacks. The resistance challenged him with out heavy weights or device. At his ultimate bodily, his doctor changed into surprised via his muscle tone, flexibility, and mobility. He might have been 80, but he felt extra wholesome, more potent, and greater lively than most people his age, way to resistance band exercises. His tale indicates you may rebuild electricity, stability, and power at any age. Resistance bands helped him defy the probabilities and stay energetic. He plans to maintain the use of them for hundreds extra healthful years.

Testimonial four (Nancy)

As a senior living alone, Nancy involved that decreased energy and mobility might possibly strain her into assisted dwelling. Simple circle of relatives obligations have become burdensome as she aged. Her daughter suggested attempting resistance bands for low-effect energy schooling she may additionally need to do from domestic. She started out out with a beginner's exercise DVD and a moderate resistance band. After a few weeks, every day sports sports like laundry, cleaning, and cooking had been a bargain much less complex. Her self warranty and stability improved from the leg and glute physical activities. Now, 18 months later, she had worked as an lousy lot as excessive resistance bands and further superior exercise exercises. At eighty one, she despite the fact that lives independently in her domestic way to normal resistance band schooling. Her center is stronger, so she has better posture and spinal stability. Her arms allow her to keep heavy gadgets once more with a bit of good fortune. The bands gave her treatment from persistent decrease back pain. Regular exercises took commitment, however the payoff has been good sized. She feels in control of her health and abilities, and resistance bands have been a huge purpose for this. They provide a clean however powerful way for seniors to assemble and maintain energy from domestic. She could not keep in mind developing antique with out this empowering device.

Testimonial five (Richard)

Like many guys his age, Richard took pleasure in his physical abilties for the duration of his existence. So, he felt defeated even as continual knee ache limited his active hobbies in his late 60s. He dreaded the concept of giving up activities like golfing, tennis, and cycling that delivered him pride. Rather than surrender himself to a sedentary way of life, he determined to fight lower again. He commenced out resistance band training on his physical therapist's advice to rebuild leg power and balance. The bands furnished a joint-nice way to exercising, and, to his wonder, he ought to see outcomes after most effective a month. His knee ache subsided, and his balance superior as his leg muscle groups reinforced. Fast in advance 5 years, and he is however faithfully doing band exercise workouts severa times in keeping with week in his domestic fitness center. Resistance bands allowed him to regain strength and mobility with out worsening his knee issues or requiring surgical procedure. Now in his 70s, he has once more to the lively pastimes he loves, way to resistance band education. His tale proves you do now not must give up hobby as you age. With self-discipline and the right tools like resistance bands, seniors can rebuild energy, control injuries, and lead energetic, fulfilling lives.

Testimonial 6 (Steven)

As a former athlete and manual laborer, it become annoying for Steven to experience his power declining in his 60s. Arthritis made weightlifting painful, so he feared his days of schooling have been over. On a chum's concept, he invested in a hard and fast of resistance bands. It end up life-converting.

The bands' flexibility provided resistance with out compressing his joints. He started out with mild tension and excessive reps to rebuild his strength foundation. Over time, he worked as much as greater difficult resistance levels by means of the use of progressing to thicker bands. Now, at 71, resistance training is still a part of his every day recurring. He does top frame art work like bicep curls and shoulder presses to preserve his fingers toned and robust. Leg physical sports like squats, lunges, and kickbacks keep him cell and beautify his stability. Picking up heavy devices or setting out to play alongside with his grandkids is simple, way to complete body energy from using resistance bands. He in no way imagined how transformational bands is probably later in existence. His spouse additionally started out using them for electricity and bone health. Resistance bands have been a whole workout changer for staying wholesome and succesful as they've elderly. He most effective wanted he had determined them faster. But it's far in no way too past because of begin energy education.

Testimonial 7 (Patricia)

As an active senior, Patricia prioritized staying healthy. So, even as she advanced again troubles that made exercising difficult in her overdue 60s, she changed into determined to discover a solution. On her chiropractor's advice, she protected resistance band sporting activities into her ordinary. The bands furnished mild resistance to beautify her again with out pressure or ache. Within months, her another time felt extensively higher and more potent. The bands have been so convenient to be used at domestic that she made them a permanent part of her everyday. Now, at seventy four, she regardless of the reality that does resistance training 3-four times in keeping with week. She rotates thru top and reduce body bodily activities to target the fundamental muscle groups and help her bones. Her stability, staying electricity, and variety of motion have advanced exceedingly. Around the residence, she movements and now not the use of a hassle, bending, lifting, and carrying items that have been as soon as too heavy. She can also stroll longer distances with out getting tired. Her treatment to take control of her fitness with resistance bands has stored her lively, independent, and entire of electricity nicely into her 70s. She is so grateful for discovering this simple tool that has empowered her to reinforce and take care of her body as she some time.

Inspiring Senior Achievements

Remaining energetic and engaged in hobbies and interests for the duration of life effects in more achievement, fitness, and properly-being for your senior years. Resistance band education empowers older adults to keep following their passions while building energy, balance, and mobility. The inspirational tales beneath exhibit seniors who have used resistance bands as a device to attain first rate accomplishments of determination, purpose, community company, and athleticism properly into their 70s, 80s, and beyond.

John, seventy eight - Grandfather Hikes Appalachian Trail

In his overdue 70s, John became although an avid hiker, playing the stunning trails near his Pennsylvania home. But he dreamed of attempting a greater epic adventure earlier than he had been given masses older – trekking the whole Appalachian Trail. In training, John commenced out out training with resistance bands at home for energy and stamina. He targeted specifically on constructing decrease body patience with squats, lunges, and thing leg lifts using the bands. After a year of everyday education, John set out to advantage his purpose, starting the over 2,000-mile Appalachian Trail in Georgia and heading north. The adventure become arduous, but John remembers his resistance band training prepared his legs and middle to address the rocky, hilly terrain. Completing the trial took 6 months. John says it come to be the maximum worthwhile revel in of his lifestyles. Resistance bands helped make it feasible through giving him the strength and stability to hike 10-15 miles each day over diverse surfaces and inclines. He hopes his story evokes others to maintain striving for large goals and understand that age by myself does now not outline what is feasible.

Betty, eighty two – Senior Bowler Rolls Perfect Game

Betty has been an avid bowler for over sixty 5 years, typically bowling in leagues given that her teenagers. At age eighty two, resistance band training is a part of her routine for keeping power, stability, and stamina to hold pursuing her lifelong ardour. Three instances in line with week, Betty does better and reduce frame sports activities the usage of resistance bands, strengthening her hands, legs, lower back, and center. She focuses in particular on her wrist, shoulder, and hip mobility and balance. On league nights, Betty arrives early to get greater flexibility work within the utilization of her bands. She credit resistance training with keeping her rolling strong in her 80s. Recently, her self-discipline paid off surprisingly whilst she completed the unusual feat of rolling a perfect three hundred-endeavor in her league. Betty says she looks as if she stays enhancing and usually mastering, and resistance bands assist make her non-prevent development possible through building energy and control. Betty hopes she can be able to encourage special seniors to keep pursuing and excelling on the pursuits they love. Setting an ambitious instance of healthy growing antique, Betty plans to compete nationally short.

Robert, eighty – Green Thumb Keeps Garden Thriving

Robert has typically loved gardening, but as he entered his 70s, tendonitis in his elbows made all the digging, lifting, and the usage of hand gear painful. He concerned he may ought to surrender gardening until he started out the usage of resistance bands to reinforce his palms, shoulders, and top decrease lower back. After several months of regular education, Robert saw a dramatic discount in his elbow tendonitis pain. Gardening have become achievable and thrilling again. Now, at eighty, Robert continues a large vegetable lawn, doing all of the planting, weeding, composting, and harvesting himself. He specializes in joint stability moves like bicep curls, upright rows, and opposite flies with resistance bands to keep his elbows, wrists, and shoulders bendy and supported. Robert moreover uses bands for lower frame training so he stays strong, carrying heavy buckets and luggage across the lawn. Resistance bands have supplied a sustainable manner for him to hold doing the activity he loves most nicely into his 80s. Robert's cute lawn continues him active and lets in offer natural produce for his own family and charity, some thing he is taking excellent satisfaction in.

Dorothy, seventy six – Volunteer Walks Dogs at Animal Shelter

Dorothy has constantly had a huge coronary heart for animals. After retiring at age sixty five, she preferred to donate her greater time to assist the animal secure haven in her network. However, chronic decrease once more issues made the bending, lifting, and taking walks required to address and stroll the dogs hard. Dorothy have emerge as keen to conquer these bodily limitations so she could pursue her volunteering passions. On her doctor's advice, she began resistance band training to gently strengthen her over again muscle mass and improve balance. She centered particularly on rotation bodily games to growth her middle mobility. Within several months of starting a ordinary band exercising ordinary, Dorothy's returned felt remarkably better and more potent. Now at seventy six, she volunteers at the animal shelter 5 days a week, on foot, feeding, and disturbing for the puppies. The resistance bands maintain her back feeling first rate and offer the stamina to be on her toes for hours. Dorothy says being involved for the animals and know-how she is developing a distinction gives her fantastic happiness and purpose. Resistance band training has allowed her to pursue a ardour later in lifestyles and provide yet again to the network.

Edward, sixty eight – Grandfather Tours America through Bike

Edward dreamed of exploring all of the small cities and backroads of rural America that he had driven with the aid of manner of for years however in no way truly skilled. At sixty 5, he provided a specialized motorcycle for multi-week tours and began resistance band schooling to situation his legs and middle for the extended daily mileage. Band carrying events like squats, lunges, thing steps, and monster walks constructed remarkable lower body power and stamina. After numerous months of diligent education, Edward released into his first multi-week solo motorcycle excursion all through South Dakota. Resistance bands gave him the leg strength to keep pedaling mile after mile. Since that first experience, Edward has biked significantly during over 30 states, immersing himself inside the culture and landscapes.

Now sixty eight, he heads out on a outstanding excursion each summer time, cycling 60-eighty miles every day over diverse terrain manner to superb conditioning from everyday resistance band exercises at home. Edward's trips have supplied wealthy life opinions and accomplishments that deliver him excellent pleasure. He hopes his trips encourage others in his age institution to pursue significant bucket list desires and understand that with training, anything is viable.

Barbara, 79 – Yoga Instructor Finds Her Calling

Barbara practiced yoga recreationally for max of her individual existence however had no thoughts of ever training. When she moved to an lively retirement network at seventy five, the citizens advised her to influence a class. Hesitant in the beginning, Barbara decided to join a teacher schooling software program. She commenced a resistance band regular to assemble power, stability, and flexibility to put together physically for demonstrating poses. Exercises like overhead presses, bicep curls, and seated rows firmed her better frame to maintain positions stably. Squats, lunges, and status leg abductions with the bands elevated hip mobility and stability for transitional movements. After completing her two hundred-hour certification, Barbara began out out training weekly yoga education to enthused citizens a great deal older than her. She credit score the resistance band schooling for giving her the self guarantee, strength, and joint stability to influence college college students successfully. Barbara loves presenting her apprehend-a way to help others revel in the identical highbrow and physical advantages she has gained from yoga for such quite a few years. She feels grateful to have observed her actual calling in her past due 70s and takes awesome satisfaction in assisting her college university college students improvement. Barbara's tale shows that you can discover new passions and skills at any age with electricity of will.

At the center of these extraordinary achievements into the 70s, 80s, and past is a dedication to staying active and constantly conditioning the frame. Resistance band education gives seniors with an effective device to construct and maintain power to keep pursuing the sports activities they love, from massive adventures like trekking the Appalachian Trail to hobbies like bowling, gardening, volunteering, swimming, biking, and yoga.

Bands assist joint fitness and mobility so seniors can live engaged in their passions pain-unfastened. They permit customizable conditioning from home to purpose muscle tissues utilized mainly sports activities activities. While ageing usually brings physical adjustments and annoying situations, resistance education can help limit losses in electricity, bone density, stability, and feature. Exercise is useful at any age to enhance health and quality of life. But extra importantly, staying active presents a experience of due to this, delight, and accomplishment.

Resistance bands empower seniors to pursue dreams and pastimes that convey pleasure and achievement every day. Consistent schooling leads to transformative consequences. But the inspirational achievements highlighted in this bankruptcy moreover display off the great spirit, stress, and abilties seniors have once they stay advocated and recollect in themselves. Their testimonies display that chronological age does now not outline what someone can acquire.

Chapter 10: Understanding Your Tools

Types and Varieties of Resistance Bands

Resistance bands are available in numerous sorts and offer a flexible technique to strength schooling, stretching, and rehabilitation physical sports. Understanding the different types and types of resistance bands is critical for deciding on the right one based totally on character fitness goals and goals. Here's a entire evaluate of the numerous kinds and forms of resistance bands:

1. Therapy Bands: These are the lightest and maximum slight styles of resistance bands.

They are normally implemented in bodily remedy and rehabilitation settings to beneficial useful resource in mild muscle strengthening and recuperation physical video video games. Therapy bands are suitable for human beings with confined mobility or individuals who are getting higher from injuries.

2. Loop Bands: Also referred to as mini bands or booty bands, loop bands form a non-stop circle with out handles. They are bendy and often used for decrease body carrying activities, which incorporates squats, leg presses, and hip abductions. Loop bands are available in particular resistance levels, making them appropriate for a huge type of customers, from beginners to superior athletes.

3. Tube Bands with Handles: These bands encompass bendy tubes with handles on every save you.

They are especially versatile and allow for a huge form of physical video video games, which consist of higher-frame, decrease-frame, and center sports. Tube bands with handles are available severa resistance stages, which can be adjusted thru changing the duration of the band or with the resource of using more than one bands concurrently.

four. Figure eight Bands: These bands are commonplace much like the variety eight and are specifically useful for focused on specific muscle organizations, together with the chest, shoulders, and palms. They provide a greater strong grip within the route of carrying sports, making them appropriate for actions that require managed resistance and balance.

5. Flat Bands: Flat resistance bands, furthermore referred to as remedy bands, are skinny, large bands without handles. They are normally used for stretching, flexibility sporting sports, and slight muscle toning.

Flat bands are available in wonderful resistance stages and are suitable for human beings searching for to enhance flexibility and mobility.

6. Layered Bands: These bands embody multiple layers of latex or rubber, providing improved resistance and sturdiness. They are designed to stand as much as immoderate levels of hysteria and are suitable for advanced power training and muscle-constructing sporting activities.

7. Fabric Bands: Fabric resistance bands are manufactured from woven material and latex, providing a more snug and non-slip grip in comparison to conventional rubber bands. These bands are excellent for users with touchy pores and pores and pores and skin or latex allergies and are generally used for each better and decrease-frame exercising exercises, similarly to stretching and mobility physical activities.

Preparing for Success

Setting Goals and Creating a Plan

Setting clean and workable health desires is essential for preserving motivation and making sure development in any exercising regimen. By developing a well-based plan, humans can establish a roadmap to achievement and effectively track their fitness journey. Here's a whole guide to setting desires and growing a plan for a a success fitness routine.

1. Define Specific Objectives: Begin with the useful resource of defining easy and unique fitness dreams, such as weight loss, muscle gain, advanced staying strength, or extra fantastic flexibility.

Make certain the ones objectives are practical and workable inside a specific time body.

2. Set Measurable Targets: Establish measurable wants to track progress efficaciously. This should embody setting intention weights, precise frame measurements, exercise frequency, or reaching sure exercising milestones. Measurable desires help in assessing improvement and staying inspired.

three. Establish a Realistic Timeline: Create a practical timeline for reaching your fitness desires. Consider your contemporary health level, way of life commitments, and any functionality traumatic conditions which could rise up. Setting an less costly timeline guarantees which you stay centered and inspired without feeling overwhelmed.

four. Create a Well-Structured Plan: Develop a complete exercise plan that consists of pretty some physical video games focused on one-of-a-kind muscle businesses. Incorporate a combination of cardiovascular sports, power schooling, and versatility wearing events to ensure a nicely-rounded and balanced health routine.

5. Gradually Increase Intensity and Duration: Plan to regularly increase the intensity and duration of your sports through the years. This modern method permits your body to comply and stops plateaus, ensuring non-stop improvement in power, persistence, and full-size fitness ranges.

6. Include Rest and Recovery Days: Integrating relaxation and restoration days into your plan is essential for muscle repair and boom.

Adequate relaxation helps prevent overtraining and decreases the chance of harm, allowing your body to get better and carry out optimally within the course of next wearing activities.

7. Monitor and Track Progress Regularly: Keep a report of your wearing sports, development, and any disturbing conditions encountered. Tracking your progress permits you to perceive regions of development, make vital modifications on your plan, and have amusing achievements alongside the way.

8. Stay Flexible and Adapt as Needed: Be open to adjusting your plan as vital to cope with any unforeseen events or modifications to your health adventure. Flexibility on your approach lets in you to stay steady and devoted to your desires, despite the fact that going through limitations or setbacks.

9. Seek Professional Guidance if Required: If you are new to health or have specific fitness troubles, keep in mind consulting a fitness trainer, bodily therapist, or healthcare professional that will help you create a custom designed and consistent exercise plan tailored for your individual goals and skills.

Upper Body Workouts

Sculpting Arms, Shoulders, and Chest

Sculpting the palms, shoulders, and chest is a key recognition for plenty people aiming to assemble better frame strength and gather a balanced body. Implementing a centered exercising habitual that emphasizes the ones muscle agencies can purpose defined and nicely-toned hands, shoulders, and chest. Here's a comprehensive manual on how to effectively sculpt these regions:

1. Warm-Up and Stretching: Begin every exercise with a dynamic heat-as a great deal as increase blood waft and prepare the muscles for workout.

Incorporate shoulder rolls, arm circles, and chest stretches to loosen up the top frame and prevent damage.

2. Arm Workouts: Incorporate numerous arm sporting events which incorporates bicep curls, tricep dips, and hammer curls to reason the biceps and triceps. Utilize one-of-a-type variations of resistance bands or weights to

offer various tiers of resistance, ensuring modern muscle development.

3. Shoulder Exercises: Include shoulder sports like shoulder presses, lateral increases, and the front will increase to goal the deltoid muscle companies. Use resistance bands or dumbbells to function resistance, specializing in controlled moves to have interaction the shoulder muscle corporations correctly.

four. Chest Workouts: Integrate chest wearing sports which includes push-ups, chest presses, and chest flies to boost and outline the chest muscle groups. Utilize resistance bands or embody variations of these wearing sports to purpose particular areas of the chest, which encompass the better, middle, and reduce chest.

5. Balanced Training Routine: Create a properly-balanced education normal that dreams all three muscle corporations correctly. Ensure that the exercise consists of a mixture of compound physical video games and remoted moves to have interaction a

couple of muscle fibers for comprehensive muscle development.

6. Progressive Overload: Gradually boom the resistance or weight used on your exercising sports to sell muscle growth and strength improvement over time.

This technique, called contemporary overload, demanding conditions the muscle tissues to comply and extend, main to huge improvements in muscle definition and energy.

7. Proper Form and Technique: Maintain proper shape and method for the duration of each exercise to efficaciously intention the desired muscle companies and prevent potential injuries. Focus on managed movements and keep away from using momentum to make certain that the focused muscle organizations are engaged at some stage in each repetition.

eight. Recovery and Rest: Allow good enough time for muscle restoration among exercising training. Adequate relaxation is vital for muscle restore and boom, so avoid overtraining and make certain which you encompass rest days into your exercising ordinary.

nine. Nutrition and Hydration: Maintain a balanced healthy dietweight-reduction plan rich in protein, healthy fat, and complex carbohydrates to manual muscle increase and restoration. Stay hydrated to promote not unusual muscle characteristic and save you muscle cramps or fatigue ultimately of workout exercises.

Chapter 11: Core Strength and Stability

Building a Solid Foundation

Building a sturdy basis in a health adventure is crucial for putting in a sturdy base and making sure prolonged-time period achievement and sustainability. Whether you're new to workout or returning after a hiatus, specializing in foundational factors is essential to carrying out ordinary health and properly-being. Here's a entire manual on a way to construct a robust foundation:

1. Assess Current Fitness Level: Begin thru assessing your cutting-edge-day health diploma and records your strengths and boundaries.

This evaluation will help you decide in which to begin and the manner to improvement successfully in your health journey.

2. Establish Clear Goals: Set unique, measurable, capacity, applicable, and time-sure (SMART) goals that align together alongside your standard fitness aspirations. Having

clear goals allows you to stay focused and inspired throughout your adventure.

three. Create a Balanced Workout Plan: Develop a properly-rounded exercising plan that includes numerous types of wearing sports, along with cardiovascular sports activities, power education, flexibility carrying sports, and stability and stability physical activities. A balanced plan guarantees that each one elements of health are addressed, fundamental to complete physical development.

4. Focus on Proper Form and Technique: Emphasize the significance of right shape and approach for the duration of sporting sports to make sure maximum pleasing muscle engagement and save you accidents. Pay hobby to posture, alignment, and respiratory techniques to maximise the effectiveness of each motion.

5. Start with Basic Exercises: Begin with fundamental bodily video video games that concentrate on essential muscle organizations

and foundational movements, inclusive of squats, lunges, push-ups, and planks. Mastering those fundamental physical games lets in set up a robust base and prepares you for additonal complex movements as you improvement.

6. Gradually Increase Intensity and Complexity: Gradually increase the depth and complexity of your bodily sports through the years to prevent plateaus and promote non-stop enhancements in energy, staying power, and traditional health. Incorporate versions and progressions of carrying occasions to assignment your frame and promote similarly improvement.

7. Prioritize Rest and Recovery: Allow ok time for relaxation and recovery among workout routines to save you overtraining and muscle fatigue. Getting sufficient sleep, training rest strategies, and incorporating rest days into your ordinary are crucial for muscle repair and boom.

8. Maintain a Healthy and Balanced Diet: Focus on ingesting a well-balanced diet regime that consists of hundreds of nutrient-dense meals, along side lean proteins, complex carbohydrates, healthy fats, and quite a few stop end result and greens. Proper vitamins helps ordinary physical fitness and complements your health efforts.

nine. Stay Consistent and Patient: Building a sturdy basis takes time and consistency. Stay affected person and devoted to your fitness everyday, and have an excellent time small achievements alongside the manner to live encouraged and devoted on your desires.

Lower Body Strength

Enhancing Legs, Glutes, and Hips

Enhancing the electricity and capability of the legs, glutes, and hips is crucial for fashionable lower frame development, balance, and mobility. By incorporating targeted sporting events that focus on these muscle corporations, human beings can decorate their decrease frame electricity, staying electricity, and easy athletic common standard overall performance. Here is a complete guide on a manner to efficaciously decorate the legs, glutes, and hips:

1. Dynamic Warm-Up: Begin each exercising session with a dynamic warmth-up that consists of leg swings, hip circles, and lunges to put together the muscle businesses for workout and growth blood float to the decrease body.

2. Leg Exercises: Incorporate some of leg wearing sports such as squats, lunges, and leg presses to target the quadriceps, hamstrings, and calf muscular tissues. Use resistance bands or weights to provide delivered resistance, frequently developing the depth to stimulate muscle boom and electricity improvement.

3. Glute Workouts: Include sports activities including hip thrusts, glute bridges, and kickbacks to in particular goal and prompt the glute muscle companies. Utilize resistance

bands or weights to feature resistance and create progressive overload, promoting glute muscle development and ordinary decrease frame balance.

4. Hip-Strengthening Exercises: Integrate hip-strengthening carrying activities like hip abductions, hip extensions, and lateral band walks to improve hip balance, flexibility, and mobility. These sports assist beautify common lower frame capability and prevent common accidents associated with prone or unstable hips.

five. Balanced Training Approach: Implement a nicely-balanced training approach that carries every bilateral and unilateral physical activities to make sure balanced muscle improvement and symmetry in the lower frame. Incorporate versions and progressions of bodily sports to constantly venture the muscle groups and promote ordinary decrease body electricity and balance.

6. Flexibility and Mobility Training: Incorporate everyday stretching and mobility

wearing activities to beautify flexibility and form of movement in the legs, glutes, and hips. Focus on dynamic stretching and foam rolling to release muscle anxiety and decorate common muscle flexibility and joint mobility.

7. Proper Form and Technique: Pay near attention to maintaining proper form and technique for the duration of every exercise to effectively goal the favored muscle groups and prevent damage. Focus on managed actions and keep away from immoderate stress at the joints to make certain that the targeted muscle mass are engaged inside the route of every repetition.

eight. Recovery and Rest: Allow good enough time for muscle healing between exercise training.

Incorporate rest days into your education agenda to sell muscle repair and increase, stopping overtraining and decreasing the danger of injury.

nine. Nutrition and Hydration: Maintain a properly-balanced eating regimen rich in vital nutrients, which includes lean proteins, complex carbohydrates, and healthful fats, to assist muscle increase and recovery. Stay hydrated to sell ordinary muscle feature and prevent muscle cramps or fatigue in the course of workout exercises.

Chapter 12: Full-Body Integration

Comprehensive Resistance Band Routines

Comprehensive resistance band workouts provide a flexible and effective technique to finish-frame exercising physical activities, allowing human beings to engage a couple of muscle corporations and benefit complete muscle improvement and firming. These routines leverage the inherent elasticity of resistance bands to create diverse stages of resistance, offering an adaptable and handy desire for electricity training, flexibility bodily sports activities, and rehabilitation. Here's a entire guide on a manner to put into effect complete resistance band sporting activities.

1. Dynamic Warm-Up: Begin each resistance band exercise with a dynamic warm-up that includes joint rotations, arm circles, and leg swings to put together the muscle agencies for exercising and increase blood go with the flow eventually of the body.

2. Upper Body Exercises: Incorporate numerous better body bodily sports, which

incorporates bicep curls, tricep extensions, shoulder presses, and chest presses, the use of resistance bands with handles or loop bands. Vary the resistance degrees to purpose awesome muscle businesses and create a entire better-frame exercising normal.

three. Core Strengthening and Stability: Integrate middle physical sports activities which incorporates status anti-rotation chops, woodchoppers, and seated Russian twists the use of resistance bands.

These physical video games interact the center muscle groups, along with the stomach muscle groups and obliques, selling center energy and balance.

four. Lower Body Workouts: Include decrease body sporting sports like squats, lunges, leg abductions, and hamstring curls the use of loop bands or resistance bands with handles. Utilize considered one among a type band resistances to successfully goal the quadriceps, hamstrings, glutes, and calves, selling lower body energy and muscle development.

5. Full-Body Integration Movements: Integrate whole-frame movements collectively with squat to overhead press, lunge with a bicep curl, and standing row to interact more than one muscle groups simultaneously.

These compound movements help decorate desired muscle coordination, stability, and realistic power.

6. Flexibility and Stretching Exercises: Conclude the resistance band normal with a sequence of stretching bodily video games that concentrate on number one muscle agencies, which include the hands, shoulders, legs, and lower again. Incorporate static and dynamic stretches to beautify flexibility, reduce muscle tension, and beautify elegant variety of motion.

Chapter 13: Intensifying Your Workouts

Intensifying your workout sports is a important approach for advancing your health adventure, hard your body, and achieving non-prevent development and improvement. By incorporating severa techniques and modifications, you could correctly growth the depth of your exercising workouts to stimulate muscle growth, enhance cardiovascular patience, and enhance conventional physical overall overall performance. Here's an entire manual at the way to heighten your exercises:

1. Progressive Overload: Gradually growth the resistance, weight, or repetitions on your strength training physical video games to undertaking your muscular tissues and promote muscle hypertrophy. Implement a established development plan to normally push your frame past its contemporary limits and stimulate muscle growth and development.

2. High-Intensity Interval Training (HIIT): Incorporate HIIT sports that contain alternating periods of excessive-depth sporting events with quick relaxation durations. This schooling technique now not top notch boosts cardiovascular endurance but furthermore will growth calorie burn and promotes fat loss, making your workout exercises greater efficient and powerful.

3. Supersets and Circuits: Combine a couple of bodily video video games into supersets or circuits to maximize the efficiency of your workout consultation. Performing bodily sports again-to-decrease lower back with out relaxation continues your heart fee increased, will growth calorie burn, and promotes muscle endurance and energy.

four. Variations in Tempo and Repetitions: Adjust the tempo of your sporting activities by way of using incorporating slow and managed moves or explosive and rapid-paced motions. Alter the sort of repetitions and devices for every exercise to venture your muscle agencies in super techniques and prevent exercising plateaus.

five. Incorporating Plyometrics: Integrate plyometric sporting activities, which includes jump squats, burpees, and area jumps, into your regular to enhance explosive power, agility, and everyday athletic typical performance. Plyometric education engages rapid-twitch muscle fibers, principal to prolonged energy and pace.

6. Utilizing Resistance Bands and Weights: Incorporate resistance bands, dumbbells, barbells, or kettlebells into your exercising workout routines to function out of doors resistance and create a extra difficult schooling environment. By growing the resistance or weight load, you can efficaciously stimulate muscle growth and decorate ordinary energy and persistence.

7. Advanced Training Techniques: Implement advanced education techniques along with drop units, pyramid units, and rest-pause sets

to push your muscle groups to their limits and sell muscle hypertrophy and power income.

These strategies introduce new worrying situations and variations, preventing your frame from adapting to the equal recurring.

8. Mind-Body Connection and Focus: Cultivate a robust thoughts-body connection at some point of sporting events by way of manner of specializing in muscle engagement, right shape, and respiration strategies. Concentrate on the centered muscle organizations and visualize the desired muscle contractions to maximize the effectiveness of each workout and optimize consequences.

9. Periodization and Recovery: Implement a based definitely periodization plan that includes periods of immoderate-intensity training, followed with the useful resource of stages of active restoration and relaxation. Balancing excessive sports with top sufficient recuperation intervals allows your frame to repair and rebuild, lowering the risk of overtraining and functionality accidents.

10. Proper Nutrition and Hydration: Fuel your frame with a well-balanced weight loss plan rich in important nutrients to beneficial resource muscle healing, restore, and growth. Stay hydrated throughout your physical games to preserve maximum amazing performance, save you muscle cramps, and sell commonplace physical nicely-being.

Tailoring Your Training

Customizing Workouts for Specific Goals

Customizing workout routines to align with specific health desires is essential for attaining targeted outcomes and maximizing ordinary exercising effectiveness. By tailoring exercise workouts to individual goals and targets, individuals can optimize their training regimens and attention on areas that require unique interest. Here is a entire guide at the manner to customise sporting occasions for precise goals.

1. Identify Specific Fitness Goals: Begin via figuring out and clarifying your unique fitness

targets, whether or now not they include weight reduction, muscle advantage, advanced cardiovascular staying power, extended flexibility, or more potent hooked up electricity. Having clean and nicely-defined goals serves as a foundational step in customizing your workout regular.

2. Targeted Exercise Selection: Select wearing events that right now motive the muscle companies or physiological systems relevant to your unique desires. For example, prioritize strength education physical activities for muscle development, include cardiovascular bodily video games for reinforcing endurance, and combine stretching and versatility physical video video games for boosting not unusual mobility.

3. Adjust Repetitions and Sets: Modify the kind of repetitions and gadgets primarily based absolutely in your preferred consequences.

For muscle building, interest on better weight masses with fewer repetitions and extra units, whilst for staying power, include lighter weights with higher repetitions and lots much less units. Adjusting the ones parameters enables tailor your exercising for your unique dreams.

4. Controlled Rest Intervals: Customize relaxation intervals among devices and physical sports primarily based completely on your desires. Longer rest intervals are suitable for energy schooling, considering muscle healing, at the same time as shorter rest durations are greater suitable for patience schooling, retaining an expanded coronary coronary heart fee, and promoting calorie burn.

five. Incorporate Specific Training Techniques: Integrate specialised education strategies alongside side isometric holds, drop devices, supersets, or plyometric carrying sports that align together with your particular fitness objectives.

These strategies can help boost up improvement, undertaking the frame, and stimulate muscle increase or patience improvement, depending for your focused dreams.

6. Adjust Resistance and Weight Loads: Modify the resistance ranges or weight loads used on your workout exercises to in form your strength and functionality level, steadily growing the resistance as you development. This approach ensures that your muscle agencies are because it must be challenged and promotes non-prevent development and boom over time.

7. Vary Exercise Modalities: Incorporate a number of workout modalities, which incorporates frame weight sporting occasions, unfastened weights, resistance bands, aerobic machines, and versatility schooling, to create a nicely-rounded exercise everyday that addresses precise factors of fitness and supports your precise dreams.

www.ingramcontent.com/pod-product-compliance
Lightning Source LLC
Chambersburg PA
CBHW060644200525
26924CB00045B/1100